T0266620

Smart and Smarter

Smart and Smarter

Enhancing Your Child's Intelligence Through Cognitive Coaching

James E. Gardner, PhD

harwood academic publishers

Australia   Canada   China   France   Germany   India
Japan   Luxembourg   Malaysia   The Netherlands
Russia   Singapore   Switzerland

Copyright © 1999 James E. Gardner. Published by license under the Harwood Academic Publishers imprint, part of The Gordon and Breach Publishing Group.

All rights reserved.

No part of this book may be reproduced or utilized in any form or by any means, electronic or mechanical, including photocopying and recording, or by any information storage or retrieval system, without permission in writing from the publisher. Printed in Singapore.

Amsteldijk 166
1st Floor
1079 LH Amsterdam
The Netherlands

British Library Cataloguing in Publication Data

Gardner, James
    Smart and smarter : enhancing your child's intelligence
    through cognitive coaching
    1. Child development   2. Education—Parent participation
    I. Title
    649. 6'8

    ISBN   90–5702–578–7

To

some very dear young friends of mine
who range from two to nine years old.
May their future, and that of all children, be filled
with people whom the philosopher John Locke called
"kind guides" to help them grow up.

Ashley *and* Megan, *my grandchildren*
Jessica *and* Lauren, *my North Carolina friends*
Andrew, Jean, Spencer *and* Maggie, *my California friends*

CONTENTS

III THE SECOND FIVE YEARS

IV PARENTS, GRANDPARENTS AND OTHER IMPORTANT PEOPLE

ACKNOWLEDGMENTS

Three people made important contributions to this book and I sincerely thank them for their considerable efforts.

The many rough edges were smoothed by the skilled editing of Carolyn Porter. Her experience and help were invaluable.

My editor Sally Cheney was always ready to offer encouragement, discuss the practical issues, and help guide the work along.

My wife Rosalind read and reread the manuscript and provided countless insights and suggestions.

I

THE NATURE OF
INTELLIGENCE

1

Enhancing Your Child's Intelligence

An introduction to cognitive coaching

This book is about how you as a parent can assist in the development of your child's intelligences. Yes, you read that correctly. There is more than one kind of intelligence. All the intelligence a child has is not fixed at birth to remain forever unchanged. Intelligence can be sharpened, focused, and enhanced. And parents can greatly assist in this enhancement.

The brain is like a muscle. Exercise through cognitive stimulation develops intellectual strength and power. Lack of such stimulation impairs development and eventually causes atrophy. Muscles are developed through exercise and the enhancement of physical skills. Likewise, the brain is stimulated by processing information—which is to say, by thinking. The more a person practices remembering, processing, synthesizing and analyzing information, the better his thinking skills will become.

As parents, we strive to meet the physical and emotional needs of our children. We guard our children's health through proper diet and exercise, introduce them to same-age social groups early, and try to provide stable, secure and loving home environments. We consider all this to be "good parenting," and it is. In some instances, however, something important is inadvertently left out of this nurturing environment. The child's intellectual growth is taken for granted. Some parents seem to assume that somehow, random events and activities—such as school, television, computer games or lessons on CD-Roms, family vacations and school field trips to interesting sites—will offer sufficient stimulation to adequately exercise the child's developing brain. Unfortunately, this is not always the case. While these activities will, of course, provide enjoyment to the child and some degree of cognitive stimulation, the development of a child's thinking abilities is too important to be left to chance, especially during that all-important first decade of life.

At present, there is strong interest in athletic programs for both boys and girls. We enhance basic physical strength, speed, and skills through a variety of training programs often initiated early in the child's life. Prodigious amounts of money and time are spent on entertainment, and special programs for the development of children in hopes that these children will grow up, become educated, and ultimately "do well" in life. It's curious, then, that so few parents and even educators seem to give sufficient time and thought to how they might help a child develop strong *thinking skills* which, hands down, will have the greatest long-term payoff in a lifetime!

If you work out, lift weights, run and jump and so on, you will soon be stronger than you were before you began your workout program. If you lift weights two or three times a week for a month or longer, you will be able to lift heavier and heavier weights up to a point. If you sprint or run long distances, especially under the tutelage of a track coach, you will soon be able to run faster and farther—up to a point. It is the *up to a point* that is being discussed here. We can improve almost any of our abilities (and help our children improve theirs) in almost any area, including cognitive skills, but only up to a point. This book does not claim that you can increase basic, innate intellectual potential—only that such potential can be *enhanced* through proper training and stimulation.

It is also important to note that though this book emphasizes the enhancement of cognitive or thinking skills, crucial basic skills such as common sense, "street smarts," a sense of humor and the ability to empathize with and understand others are also important aspects of intelligence which will be woven into our program.

Good parents have their child's best interests at heart. They would most likely help their child develop ability in any area, especially in thinking skills, if they could. Yet, few parents seem to embark on any kind of active and consistent cognitive coaching type of program. Perhaps they feel that schools will bear this responsibility even though this will unfortunately not be the case. Or, parents may have simply never given the matter much thought. Some may have heard about cognitive stimulation but may not know how to develop such a program for their child.

In the early years, parents and grandparents or others who can give interesting and focused one-to-one time to a child are by far the most important and most effective tutors. Until we arrive at chapter 15, which speaks specifically about grandparents, the word "parents" will stand for the actual parents, grandparents, older siblings, or any interested adult who is in close contact with the child. All that parents need in order to generate a good cognitive stimulation program is the willingness to spend some individual time with their child, coupled with some basic ideas about cognitive enhancement during the all-important early years. The ideas are in this book. The motivation has to come from you.

THE PREMISE

The premise here is simple. It involves the belief that it is better for a child to be bright, alert, cognitively capable, and very competent in various intellectual, social, artistic and athletic domains than not. We want our children to be good thinkers, exercise good judgment, do well academically, have positive self-esteem, and have confidence in their own ability to think clearly and to solve problems. We want our children to be smart. And by that we mean bright with good street sense as well as intellectual or book smarts. And by that we mean *intelligent*.

We also want our children to be well-educated and, when grown, to engage in emotionally and financially rewarding careers. Cognitive coaching enhances educational achievement because it enhances thinking skills. The importance of education, in addition to its intrinsic rewards, is underscored by the economist, James Flanigan, who states that "... by far the biggest differentials in wages are accounted for by education. A high school dropout earns $306 a week on average, while high school graduates earn $426 a week and college graduates $704 a week. If the person gets a graduate degree, he or she can look for $1,200 to $1,900 a week."[1]

In sports, coaches want athletes who are strong and fast. These attributes are considered to be building blocks from which other skills may be developed. Coaches now want athletes who are also bright. National Football League teams routinely administer IQ tests in addition to the usual tests of speed and strength prior to the player draft.[2]

Although each of us is born with limitations on our maximum strength and speed, most of us don't work out hard enough or long enough to reach these limits. As a consequence, most of us are not as fast or as strong as we could be. It's exactly the same with intelligence.

AN IMPORTANT WARNING

Although we are going to be talking at some length about the enhancement of your child's thinking skills through cognitive coaching, it is *extremely* important to understand that this is not to be done in some formal or high-pressure way! This entire program should be implemented in an easy way and at an enjoyable pace for both parent and child. It is a kind of daily learning program made up of bits and pieces from everyday life. Pressuring a young child to "learn" can block his desire for learning and, worse, cause him to want to avoid spending time with the parent or "instructor." The famous educator, John Holt, showed us the results of the fear of failure among elementary school age children. As the child becomes fearful and tries to come up with a "right answer," her ability to think clearly and rationally actually declines.[3] The cognitive coaching approach advocated here is not like a traditional tutoring session. The parent provides intellectual stimulation through conversation, reading and thinking out loud, playing games and doing many other activities which we will be discussing. But it must be done carefully and caringly and *without pressure*!

WHAT IS INTELLIGENCE?

Intelligence is the ability to learn, remember, and constructively generalize the learned behavior from one activity to another; to creatively, adaptively and effectively problem-solve; to be able to think vicariously and to use and manipulate symbols; and to have the imaginative capacity for creating new thoughts or ideas based on previously learned material.

Traditional thought equates intelligence with having good verbal or math skills. Although verbal and math abilities are indeed critically important in the modern world, there are other important domains of intellectual functioning as well. These other domains involve social, spatial, artistic, musical, artistic, athletic and other intellectual competencies. Many researchers in the field of intelligence have conceptualized overall intelligence as stemming from a general intellectual reservoir or g factor.

Those who believe in theories of multiple intelligence tend to play down the g factor and do not necessarily agree that being bright or skilled in one area correlates with having strengths in other areas. Certainly, the skilled editor of a magazine may not necessarily play the violin very well or at all, though she can write forcefully and edit well. Howard Gardner, a Harvard neuropsychologist, has been a major proponent of the concept of multiple intelligences. Gardner argues for the existence of an "intelligence" in areas such as linguistic, musical, logical-mathematical, spatial, bodily-kinesthetic and personal.[4]

Controversy surrounds Gardner's theory. The majority of psychologists researching the nature of intelligence are convinced that a g factor underpins all other factors. It is noted by some psychologists that the various domains Gardner puts forward as intelligences are essentially skill areas, which are offshoots of a fundamental intelligence—the g factor.

The debate regarding what kind of intelligence or intelligences we possess will go on. However, there is virtually complete agreement among experts that verbal, rational, logical, analytical thinking—when aided and abetted by intuitive or right-brained thinking, swift information processing systems in the auditory and visual realms, and good street smarts—is a prescription for success in the academic realm and in the workforce of the future.

Intelligence has been defined, somewhat facetiously, as that which intelligence tests measure. This kind of remark is about as accurate as calling running speed that which stopwatches measure. No matter how we measure or define it, most of us recognize intelligent behavior (or running speed) when we see it. Not only do we recognize intelligence, we want our kids to have as much of it as possible. Everyday examples of our children doing something that we label "bright" or "clever" abound. The very verbal VCR-using two-year old, the problem-solving puzzle-constructing four-year old, the already-reading-well six-year old, the philosophical-humorous eight-year old, and the ten-year old computer whiz kids who take Windows 95 in stride and write their own programs for computer games—these are children we see in daily life.

We know that such children are smart, their parents know they are smart, and their teachers know they are smart. Presumably, their peers see them as smart, too. Some children just seem to think and do things in more effective ways than others. These are the intelligent children, the children who have a head start on the future.

An informal answer to the question "What is intelligence?" might simply note that intelligent behavior is that which works well in a given situation while concomitantly considering the consequences of that behavior. The toddler who learns to open the closet door and un-lock the top of his playtoy box, the school age child who learns to link sounds and symbols and acquires the ability to read, and the older child who considers bus routes and starting times at the ball park are all engaged in purposeful, directed, intelligent behaviors. All humans think, of course, but the higher the level of thinking skills in any given situation, the more effective will be the individual's behavior.

ISN'T INTELLIGENCE FIXED AT BIRTH?

Aren't people either born with smarts or not? Isn't thinking ability, whether high-level or low-level, built into the hardwiring of a per-son's brain right from the start? If there is room for development through training and stimulation, what is the limit? How much boost could we expect from a cognitive stimulation program?

About half of our intelligence is considered to be fixed at birth—set by the genes, as it were. The other half is malleable, so our intelligence can be developed depending upon what does or does not happen to us during our formative years. It is safe to say that most of us do not come close to reaching the full potential of our intelligence, even though we may have been provided with the "usual" cognitive stimu-lation inherent in good schools and a middle-class background. Sadly, a large number of children living in impoverished environ-ments and/or abusive situations do not even come close to the full development of their intellectual powers. These are stunted children, and they represent an unfortunate waste for themselves and to society.

It is also a waste when children from so-called "good homes" are not stimulated toward the enhancement of their cognitive skills. In today's busy world, children tend to be provided with high-tech toys such as computers, which are touted as stimulating the child's think-ing abilities. Prior to providing the child with computer technology, middle-class parents also participate with their children in early childhood programs such as Mommy and Me, Gymboree, and pre-school. In an ironic twist, many of these young children must also spend time in daycare centers or with housekeepers while both par-ents work in order to pay for these programs and other accout-erments of the "good life."

AT BIRTH, INTELLIGENCE IS ONLY A POTENTIAL

At birth, a child's ultimate level of intelligence is more a *potential* than a measurable or observable entity. Intelligence is not a fixed and immutable fact of life. The number of neurons present in the human brain is some ten billion, with a typical neuron making thousands of connections with other cells through synapses. The total number of synaptical connections in the brain is something like ten trillion.[5] If there is insufficient stimulation of the brain in the early years, a permanent limit is placed on the number of synapses, and hence, on intellectual potential. In other words, without an adequate and appropriate amount of stimulation which fosters connections between brain cells, there is a limit on the development of intelligence.

A famous experiment illustrates the point. Neuropsychologists at the University of California at Berkeley placed a group of young rats in a "high stimulation" environment consisting of all sorts of rat toys and mazes on which they could climb, jump about and crawl through. Another group was reared in a "low stimulation" environment which consisted of a virtually bare environment with just food and water. Later, when examined, the animals from the high-stimulation environment were found to have significantly heavier brains with more and denser neural connections.[6]

The stimulation provided by early childhood education programs such as Headstart has been shown to result in measurable gains in the intelligence of the children involved.[7] The Headstart environment, using much cognitive stimulation, results in measurable differences in thinking skills for these students.

HOW IS INTELLIGENCE MEASURED?

Intelligence, thinking skills, and cognitive capacity are, for our purposes, essentially similar. Intelligence is inferred from such things as:

- Observations of the child's problem-solving behavior in various circumstances
- School grades and other assessments of academic performance
- IQ tests

School grades and academic achievement tests are often used by educators and parents to estimate a child's intelligence. However, because of factors such as differences in motivation and environment, these are not perfect estimators. The highly motivated "grind" who spends many hours a day studying will often obtain better grades than the student who eschews studying, and instead spends much time playing or being a couch potato watching TV. However, the student who devotes a lot of time to homework and test preparation will not necessarily score the highest on standardized achievement tests such as the Stanford Achievement Test or the Educational Records Bureau test battery. The brighter student who reads extensively might score well on the verbal portions of these tests, but not have sufficient motivation or perseverance to maintain the type of regular study schedule necessary to obtain good grades.

Well-constructed IQ tests such as the Wechsler Intelligence Scale for Children, 3rd Edition (WISC-III) are very good at estimating certain aspects of a child's intelligence.[8] This test is effective in approximating, in particular, a child's verbal versus non-verbal cognitive skills and providing a Verbal IQ, a Performance IQ and a Full Scale IQ score. The latter is considered to be a reasonably good index of an individual's overall level of intellectual functioning. The WISC-III also provides the examiner (usually a clinical psychologist or school psychologist) with a great deal of information based on its subtests. IQ tests such as the WISC-III—when combined with observational data in school or elsewhere, background data from home or other sources, and examined in conjunction with the child's performance on school tests and projects—provide a sound basis for judging the child's cognitive capacities in a number of areas. It can also be helpful in planning for her education. The IQ test is very useful as a quick method for obtaining a great deal of valuable information about the child's intellectual potential as well as possible underlying learning disabilities which may be present.

AREN'T OTHER DIMENSIONS OF A PERSON ALSO IMPORTANT?

Other dimensions of an individual are, of course, very important. The concept of an "emotional intelligence" has generated much recent interest.[9] The ability to relate well to others, to empathize, to offer honesty and friendship to others, and so on are important. I believe that these skills, like cognitive skills, are teachable. These matters are discussed in this book as part of the general enhancement of thinking skills.

Motivation or drive is extremely important in almost any area of endeavor. Individuals with high intelligence but low drive are not choosing to make maximum use of their gifts. On the other hand, a highly motivated individual with average intelligence may accomplish great things. It has been said that "genius is as genius does," meaning that high IQ scores are worthless if nothing is done with all that intellectual horsepower.

An agreeable personality is a critically important dimension. Some highly intelligent people cannot manage to get along well with others and are simply disagreeable, miserable human beings. There are others of average intelligence who are socially adept, manifest a good sense of humor, and have street smarts. Shakespeare's Iago was presented as highly intelligent, though a trouble-making sociopathic personality. We are all aware of doctors, lawyers, accountants, politicians, and others who are bright, successful and well-educated, but who lack kindness and compassion.

Although having good cognitive skills do not in and of themselves make someone a decent person, this should not preclude us from enhancing such skills to every extent possible. However, we should also always help our children develop traits such as honesty, decency, compassion and kindness. In fact, once the parent understands cognitive coaching, "conscience coaching," can be easily figured out and implemented.

DON'T SCHOOLS DEVELOP THINKING SKILLS FOR OUR KIDS?

Schooling is very important—we are not trying to replace your child's school experience. Cognitive coaching is an add-on, if you will, something you do as a kind of personalized enrichment program. Although school is and will continue to be a very important experience for our children as they grow up, school is not the beginning and end of their cognitive, social or emotional development. From a cognitive development standpoint, today's public schools for the most part tend to teach to the average student. In tomorrow's world, average street smarts and average book smarts are not likely to be sufficient. There is just too much competition out there from too many people and many of them are very bright. It seems likely that your child will need to be able to function in an above average manner in several of the intellectual areas discussed in this book in order to be successful in the future.

Some parents feel that private school is the answer. However, few parents can afford the high tuitions (one Los Angeles private school's tuition for kindergarten is over $10,000 per year, with this amount increasing through the upper grade levels). But even the expensive and exclusive private schools are no panacea, especially since most schools still use a general curriculum and don't give special attention to individual students. If your child is in private school, she will still be better off with additional intellectual stimulation from her parents in areas involving thinking, social skills and value judgments.

Indeed, there has been a "dumbing down" of many schools, including some private schools, in order to accommodate the often shoddy and half-baked thinking skills of so many of the students. Television, that great anesthetist, seems to have numbed many brains, because it is a passive medium. The Scholastic Aptitude Test (SAT) has had to be "recentered" at a lower level in order to adjust for the continuing downward drift in our children's thinking/knowledge skills.[10] Readers and thinkers with good math skills are going to be in demand and in command in tomorrow's world.

IS THERE A "BEST TIME" IN A CHILD'S LIFE FOR THE ENHANCEMENT OF INTELLIGENCE?

The prime time for intellectual/social/personal development in all domains is during the first decade of life, with the early years being the most important. The human brain is very malleable during this time. From birth through the period up to puberty, the brain is most receptive to—and needs the most—cognitive stimulation. As we have seen, young rats who received more stimulation in an enriched environment showed significant brain growth, but even adult animals showed dramatically increased abilities in mazes testing agility and intelligence when appropriate cognitive stimulation had been provided.[11] Cognitive stimulation appears to be important at all age levels.

CHILDREN HAVE NO VOTE

Children have absolutely no say about whether or not their parents will choose to enhance their cognitive potential. The child cannot decide on his own that he will develop better skills in thinking, remembering, processing and sorting information, range of vocabulary and strong perceptual functioning. He does not possess the ability to know about and implement a program of cognitive coaching.

He is at the mercy of parents, teachers, and other caretakers with respect to material which might stimulate intellectual capacity. Television, arcade games, and school are the poor engines which cannot generate superior intellectual enhancement of children in our society. Parents, in general, play an amazingly small part in this endeavor except to donate the genetic background and room and board. For example, Richard Louv in *Childhood's Future* cites a 1988 study revealing that "...*the average working parent spends (only) thirty seconds per day in meaningful conversation with his or her children.*" However, as parents become more aware of the positive gains which are to be derived from time spent in cognitive coaching, or even just "hanging out" with their kids, we are likely to see more parents devoting more individual time to their children.

The amount of simple "time spent" in easy and interesting activities with a child is truly important for the child's development. There can be no "quality time" unless there is "quantity time." And all activities need not center on the child. Children learn much by observing what and how a parent goes about her daily activities. If you value reading and want your child to grow up to be a reader, turn off the TV and read a book for your own pleasure. We serve as role models for our children in many subtle but important ways.

THE POSITIVE SIDE-EFFECTS OF COGNITIVE COACHING

This book, as we have discussed, is about enhancing your child's intelligence. Again, intelligence is meant in the broadest sense and includes social intelligence, personal sensivity, empathy, and awareness of conscience and values. It is about helping your child attain optimal cognitive development. Our society has moved from agrarian to industrial to technical to electronic. The premium now is placed on thinking skills rather than physical strength. Whether we like it or not, a quick, well-trained mind has become highly desirable now and in the foreseeable future.

Regardless of the sophistication of our cognitive coaching techniques, however, we repeat that we cannot generate *more* intellectual capacity than an individual innately possesses. It is important that it be understood that we are not talking about increasing intelligence in some mystical and remarkable manner, but instead, we are discussing enhancing the intellectual potential with which the child was born. Since parents cannot be assured of either the kind or the degree of cognitive stimulation which might or might not be provided by preschool or school, they will have to shoulder the pleasant burden of much of this task themselves.

The "task," incidentally, is not overly difficult or complex. It is generally quite enjoyable. If you approach the job with a *good attitude* and are *imaginative* and *not pushy*, the side effects of a cognitive coaching program can be:

- A more positive relationship between you and your child.

- A better understanding of how children think and of how your child best thinks and learns.

- A more informed appraisal on your part of what kind of school or other educational program might best fit your child's needs.

- A greater awareness on your part of what school and computers do or do not offer your child in terms of cognitive stimulation.

In closing this chapter, I return to John Holt's thoughts on children's learning. Holt said that "...vivid, vital pleasurable experiences are easiest to remember...memory works better when unforced—it is not a mule that can be made to walk by beating it...when we make children afraid we stop learning dead in its tracks."[12]

We want our children to enjoy thinking and learning. And we most assuredly do not want them to become negatively conditioned to learning because of parental pressure. Be an easy, pleasant coach; have fun with your child and enjoy your role as coach.

NOTES

1. Flanigan, James. "Income and Education," *Los Angeles Times*, June 18, 1995.
2. Plashke, Bill and Almond, Elliott. "Has the NFL Draft Become A Thinking Man's Game?" *Los Angeles Times*, April 21, 1995.
3. Holt, John. *How Children Fail*. New York: Delta, 1964.
4. Gardner, Howard. *Frames of Mind*. New York: Penguin. 1979.
5. Russell, Peter. *The Brain Book*. New York: Penguin. 1979.
6. Krech, D., Rosenzweig, M.R., and Bennett, E.L., "Environmental impoverishment, social isolation and changes in brain chemistry and anatomy." *Physiological Behavior*, 1, 1966. pp. 99–109.
7. Besharov, Douglas. *The Bell Curve Debate*. Russell Jacoby and Naomi Glauberman (Eds) New York: Random House Times Books. 1995. p. 361.

8. Wechsler, David. Wechsler Intelligence Scale for Children—3rd Edition. San Diego: Harcourt Brace Jovanovitch. 1991.
9. Goleman, Daniel. *Emotional Intelligence*. New York: Bantam, 1995.
10. Steward, Donald. "New SATs for a new kind of student," *Wall Street Journal*, October 4, 1995.
11. Hotz, Robert. "Battle For Hearts and Minds," *Los Angeles Times*, April 3, 1997.
12. Holt, John. *How Children Learn*. New York: Pitman. 1967.

2

The Distribution of Intelligence

When determining levels of intelligence of various groups of people, it appears that intelligence, like other human attributes such as height and weight, is distributed in the pattern of a bell-shaped curve. Most people fall somewhere in the middle of the curve, fewer on the ends, and even fewer at the extreme tails of the curve. To illustrate, let's assume that an intelligence (IQ) test has been administered to a great many children in a particular town. If these children were then asked to line up on the football field according to a coded IQ number assigned to each, a pattern would take form. If the fifty-yard line was equated with an IQ score of 100, we would find more children lined up on that yard line than on any other. Each yardage marker away from the fifty-yard line, on either side, will find fewer and fewer children in the line. By the time we reached the goal lines on either side, there would be, perhaps, only one child on each goal line. One of these children would have a very high IQ (at the 99 percentile or higher) and the other child a very low IQ (at the 1 percentile or lower).

If we observed the field from above, the pattern would show the majority of children in the middle of the field, with the numbers declining as we near each goal line. This is the picture of the normal bell shaped curve as illustrated in Figure 1.

Why is intelligence distributed in this manner? For the same reason that height or weight, speed or strength, sense of humor, or any other human trait is distributed in the same way. The "Law of Large Numbers" statistically assures that as you measure certain traits in any large population, the distribution smoothes toward one resembling a bell-shaped curve. However, with respect to intelligence, this does not imply that any given child's position is immutably fixed and unchangeable.

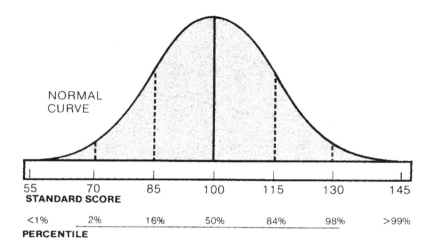

NORMAL
CURVE

55	70	85	100	115	130	145

STANDARD SCORE

| <1% | 2% | 16% | 50% | 84% | 98% | >99% |

PERCENTILE

Figure 1   Intelligence distribution

Even though the distribution may be relatively fixed for the physical variable of height, it is not necessarily fixed with respect to weight, running speed, or strength or intelligence. These attributes can be altered through training, and an individual may, figuratively speaking, move up or down the field to a different yard marker, depending on training or lack of it through the years.

A child may start out, let us say, with a placement on the plus or minus side of the fifty-yard line (letting plus (+) be above-average or higher intelligence and minus (–) stand for lower or under 100 IQ). Let's place child A slightly on the plus side at birth. This hypothetical child is then subjected in her early years to a home environment in which there is spousal abuse, the parents and the older children use drugs daily, chaos is commonplace and normal intellectual stimulation and development are virtually impossible. This unfortunate child, then, would be likely to drift down from her place above the fifty yard line, cross this marker at some point, and continue drifting downward into the negative markers. This child is, in effect, "losing IQ." This sad scenario is an unfortunate fact of life for many children in our country. These children never reach their intellectual or personal potential. Their loss is a loss for all of us since every society in the modern world needs the intellectual power of all of its citizens.

A happier scenario exists when a fifty-yard line child at birth receives average intellectual stimulation within a more or less "normal" daily environment, with normal being defined as non-abusive, reasonably caring, and having school, books, conversation and other adequate stimulation. This child will do no worse than hold her place on the fifty-yard line, and perhaps will move up farther into the positive side of the field depending upon the interests she develops, teachers she may have over time, and stimulation provided by her parents.

An even better scenario, of course, would occur if the child is well into the positive side of the field at birth—the twenty-yard line, let's say—and is provided with adequate or even superior stimulation in the form of words, ideas, books, schooling, participation in extracurricular activities, camps and vacations and good parental involvement. Our twenty-yard line child is likely not only to hold his place on that marker but probably move up a bit as well, possibly to the fifteen- or even ten-yard line.

Why not to the goal line? Or, at least the one- or two-yard line? Recall the ceiling effect. No matter what, there is no reason to believe that we can develop any individual past his biological limits. This is so in terms of speed and strength, as well as in terms of intelligence. It is likely that the child who starts on the twenty-yard line can move up some of the way toward the five- or ten-yard line, but a limit will always be reached.

But, isn't the child who is virtually born with the capacity for placement on the twenty-yard line already bright enough? Won't this child, being in the top 10 percent or so of intelligence nationwide, tend to do very well in most things he attempts? Yes, of course he will. When a child is at this level, parents could actually afford to be somewhat sanguine about their child's further intellectual development. This is because many very bright children are virtual learning machines. They are autodidacts, actively seeking more intellectual stimulation. Such a child will respond well to any additional intellectual stimulation a parent provides. Even so, the child may not move up a great deal in terms of our yardage marker illustration. Again, this is because of the fixed limits beyond which we cannot go. The nearer one is to his fixed limit in any field of human activity, the less room there is for upward movement.

However, most of us, including our children, function somewhere in the middle of the field. In general, there is probably considerable room for improving our thinking skills. And, for the child in his first decade of life, there is ample reason to believe that not only is there considerable room for gaining greater intellectual powers, but that this is the easiest and best time for such gains to take place. Even so, as we've stated, someone must take the lead in providing the additional stimulation necessary for the child to positively alter his position in the distribution.

Mother Nature is not a bigot with respect to the distribution of intelligence. There are individuals of very high, average, and very low intellectual capacity among all groups of people. There is reason to believe that children of all groups, regardless of where they stand in the initial distribution of intelligence (their place on the yardage marker, as it were), would benefit from enrichment activities within a program of early cognitive stimulation. Good cognitive skills need to be developed early in order that the child is well-prepared to think powerfully, efficiently and effectively when the need arises.

3

How Intelligence is Measured

Intelligence, as an extremely valuable commodity, has probably been assessed or evaluated in some manner since the earliest of times. It was undoubtedly very useful for the elders to carefully evaluate who among the children in a tribe or clan would make the best hunters, medicine men or women, fighters or builders and so on and begin to channel their development at an early age.

Polynesian boys in the time of the Pacific migrations were selected early with respect to skills in sailing and carefully apprenticed in the art of moving their boats over great distances from one island to another, guided by stars and the feel of the currents.[1] We can easily imagine the Romans selecting young people with administrative intelligence to govern their far-flung empire; the Egyptians selecting and training bright young boys with geometric skills to advance their pyramid and other building projects; or the ancient Japanese selecting and training the next generation of samurai warriors.

It was not until the early part of the 20th century, however, that the first quantification of the selection for intelligence took place. In 1905, French psychologists Alfred Binet and Theodore Simon devised the first scale of intelligence for schoolchildren.[2] A scale of age norms, later called Mental Ages, was developed. The notion of "IQ" was born when the concept of Mental Age divided by Chronological Age yielding an Intelligence Quotient was developed.

In this book, the terms IQ, intelligence, and cognitive skills are used more or less interchangeably. Technically, however, an IQ is a number generated by the child's performance on an intelligence test. The

21

assumption is that the number, the IQ, reflects some form or forms of intelligence. Intelligence, then, is a combination of various cognitive or thinking skills. IQ represents a particular score on a standardized intelligence test, while intelligence or cognitive skills may be inferred either from the IQ score or from a child's observable behaviors.

The Polynesian sailor mentioned earlier may, for instance, have had remarkable "intelligence" because of his ability to cross vast stretches of ocean. This intelligence involved various cognitive or thinking skills which may have operated almost subliminally to compute time, current, distance and wind. However, unless this boy were long exposed to schools such as we have in our culture, his score on an IQ test, even one given in his own language, may not rate him as outstanding. In fact, our test could possibly record his intelligence as only average, or even below average. On the other hand, few in our culture could possibly exhibit his type of visual-spatial-kinesthetic intelligence on the water.

In other words, IQ tests are culture-bound. We know this and accept it. But, because our children are growing up in this North American culture, not that of the Polynesian or Eskimo or Bushman or any other, it is desirable that they develop an "IQ test" kind of intelligence as well as other talents or intelligences that suit our culture. What does an IQ score tell us?

In his book on intelligence testing, the educational psychologist Alan Kaufman notes, "The IQ does not reflect a global summation of the brain's capabilities and is certainly not an index of genetic potential, but *it does predict school achievement effectively.*[3] Interestingly, IQ, as an estimate of overall or global intelligence, is a good predictor of many more things than just school achievement. As a very practical example, the IQ score turns out to be the best predictor of adult job performance, winning out over other factors such as educational background, grades, the interview, resume reviews or reference checks.[4]

If we add to the mix some reasonably accurate and valid estimates of cognitive strengths and types of thinking derived from an IQ test and/or derived from direct observations of the child's behavior, we can perceive that a "high IQ" is a positive in our society. We can also perceive that being able to think quickly, thinking thoroughly through a problem, being street smart, having the ability to articulate one's thoughts by the spoken or written word, and being able to move easily in the digitalized world of the internet are all tremendously useful skills. Since no one is born with these skills fully in place, we look to parents and others to help the child develop them.

At the present time, the measurement of intelligence through test-ing—as opposed to direct observation of some particular behaviors which are considered "smart" or adaptive—is largely carried out through administration of one of several IQ tests, such as:

- The Wechsler Intelligence Scale for Children-III (WISC-III) for children age six through sixteen.

- The Wechsler Preschool and Primary Scales of Intelligence (WPPSI) for children under age six.

- The Stanford-Binet Intelligence Scales-4th Edition used from preschool ages through high school and beyond.

There are also other tests which help estimate intelligence which are less verbal, such as:

- The Peabody Picture Vocabulary Test.

- The Woodcock-Johnson Tests of Cognitive Abilities-Revised.

All tests mentioned here are individually administered, and all but the Peabody require an hour or more to administer. There are various less reliable and valid group tests used by schools. Interpretation of group tests tends to be difficult, since they all require reading ability. Unfortunately, not all children, even though of average or above-average intelligence can read well, and some—those who are dys-lexic, for instance—can hardly read at all.

By the time a child takes one of the above IQ tests (assuming she ever does) she will have experienced many things and many people. She will doubtless have learned many social skills and other vital skills, such as how to walk and talk and feed herself, as well as how to think about things symbolically (for example, playing dress-up with mother's clothes; playing at being a fire fighter; imagining oneself as a ballet dancer, and so on). This kind of thinking and more would be evident even if the IQ test was administered at age two or three years. How-ever, testing a child this young is rare. In general, intelligence tests administered to infants and very young children are used either for research purposes to study how infants respond, or because a doctor suspects some degree of brain damage or severe developmental delay.

Sometimes, parents request the administration of an IQ test for a young child because they want to plan for future schooling or because of suspected school learning difficulties. If the latter is the case, tests for underlying perceptual dysfunctions as well as tests which evaluate the child's emotional status should also be administered.

As we have said, intelligence is not a single entity. An individual can have different strengths in various areas. The following different "domains" of intelligence are important building blocks for overall good thinking skills:

- Abstract reasoning ability

- Math computational ability

- A broad general fund of information

- A good vocabulary

- A good understanding of one's environment

- The ability to focus attention

In Part III we will discuss ways to enrich your child's cognitive skills through use of concepts in the domains of intelligence listed above and below. The intellectual areas noted above involve, for the most part, left-brain or verbal skills. The areas listed below involve right-brain or non-verbal domains of intelligence which are also important in school and in daily life.

- The ability to keenly discriminate small details

- The quick perception of cause-effect sequences

- The ability to grasp the overall conceptual picture

- The capacity to deal with part-whole or spatial relations

- The use of eye-hand dexterity and visual memory

- The ability to focus and refocus attention

Since it may not be intuitively obvious why all these aspects of cognition and perception are important, let's take a closer look at just one of them—the ability to discriminate small details.

The ability to discriminate or quickly perceive small details may be useful in many different circumstances. Academically, such an ability would probably be very useful in terms of following directions in class or on homework, checking out a barometric pressure readout or other precise formulation, following the plus or minus or times signs in math, and so on. Socially, this skill is useful in terms of "reading" the nuances of the expressions of others.

A WARNING ABOUT IQ TEST RESULTS

If your child should ever take an individual IQ test, it is likely that the test will be the widely-used and well-constructed Wechsler Intelligence Test for Children—Third Edition (WISC-III). The following comments are specific to the WISC-III but are relevant to all IQ test scores.

The principal reason why the Full Scale IQ score of the WISC-III—or even the more specific Verbal or Performance IQ scores—do not truly do justice to any individual child is that the same score can be reached by vastly different sets of subtest scores. For example, a child may obtain a Verbal IQ score of, say, 120 and a Performance IQ score of only 80, resulting in a Full Scale IQ estimate of 100, exactly in the average range. But the 120 score would place the child in the top 10 percent intellectually with the 80 IQ score being in the lower 10 percent. The Full Scale IQ score of 100 is, of course, exactly at the 50 percent level, but this is misleading because of the great disparity between the Verbal and Performance scores, from which the Full Scale IQ is derived. In this case, we would know that the child's verbal skills are very strong, but the deficits in the non-verbal areas may impair fluid academic functioning in areas involving the need to discriminate fine details, grasp part-whole relations, perceive cause-effect sequences, and so on. Such a child, though very bright verbally, might well be highly frustrated on various academic tasks.

There are many combinations which can take place among the subtest scores, causing the subtest analysis, not the IQ scores, to be the critically important aspect of an IQ test such as the WISC-III. The subtests can yield much valuable information with respect to an individual's intellectual strengths and weaknesses, with this information going well beyond the listing of IQ scores. If your child has taken a WISC-III or any other IQ test at school, be sure that it is interpreted only by a psychologist experienced with the meaning of this material.

In closing this chapter, we note that the school-age child has been developing and refining his genetic/biological basis for intellectual functioning for many years. The more enriched an environment this development has taken place in, the greater the child's cognitive capacities and skills will be, up to that indefinable point at which nurture (the environment) bumps into the ceiling imposed by nature (the genetic makeup).

In the old days, many parents relied heavily on schools to stimulate and enrich their children's minds. This may have been adequate in the past but, as we've said, it's no longer an option. In the next chapter, we examine the problems of the schools.

NOTES

1. Gladwin, T. *East Is A Big Bird: navigation and logic on Puluwat Atoll.* Cambridge, Mass.: Harvard University Press, 1970.
2. Boring, Edwin. *A History of Experimental Psychology.* New York: Appleton-Centruy-Crofts, 1950. pp. 573–574.
3. Kaufman, Alan. *Intelligent Testing With the WISC-R.* New York: Wiley, 1979. p. 9.
4. Gottfredson, Linda. "Reconsidering Fairness: a matter of social and ethical priorities," *Journal of Vocational Behavior*, 33, 1988. pp. 293–319.

4

The Dumbing Down of Schools

The two primary educational tasks of today's public schools is to first teach basic academic skills at the elementary level, and to then branch out to teach higher level academic skills at the middle and senior high school levels. In a multi-ethnic, multilingual society such as ours, this is quite a task in and of itself. And to add to their responsibility, the schools are often expected to provide social services such as counseling, nutritional, and remedial programs. Communities also look to schools to provide an oasis of relative safety and calm in neighborhoods awash with chaos and violence.

Americans have not always expected so much from their schools. When this country was young, schools were founded in large measure because "…schooling was intended to cultivate a respect for the laws of the theocratic state and the sanctity of property."[1] In an essentially Protestant country at the time, the "three Rs" were important for religious and economic reasons. It was further assumed that schooling "…would contribute to a person's economic and social usefulness by cultivating literacy, resourcefulness, enterprise, punctuality, and thrift."

Although it was considered important for each person to learn to read and to perform rudimentary mathematical calculations, children were nevertheless seasonally removed from school when they were needed as "hands" for the family farm. Clearly and understandably, survival of the family and, by extension, the township in which the family lived, had precedence over school attendance.

It was not until the twentieth century that school attendance began to be regarded as important for all children. The elementary schools were extended into middle and high schools. By 1918, the law in thirty states specified full-time attendance until age sixteen.[2] Even so, for the majority, obtaining a high school or college degree was more a rarity than the norm in those days.

After World War II, however, earning a high school degree became more important and eventually became almost universally expected. Today, the lack of a high school diploma has become a stigma of some consequence. Only about fifteen percent of the population do not attain a high school degree or equivalent at the present time. However, most readers of this book will want at least a college degree for their youngster, and perhaps desire post-graduate work that will lead to an advanced degree.

It is unlikely, of course, that all parents who want their children to attend Harvard Law School are going to see that dream realized. Even if all of our children were bright and studious enough to qualify for Yale, Stanford or the University of California, Berkeley (or their equivalents among many other fine universities), the reality is that there are insufficient openings in the top schools for the number of applicants. Another reality, perhaps somewhat less palatable, is that very few students intellectually qualify for top universities, and many are not even intellectually or academically well-suited for far less competitive slots at state universities.

It is very difficult to know how far any given student might go academically if provided with sufficient educational enrichment starting in the first decade of life and continuing through high school. It is obvious that a student with insufficient intellectual enrichment is much less likely to go as far academically as is his counterpart who received such stimulation, assuming their basic intelligence was initially somewhere near the same range.

Unfortunately, our educational system cannot be relied upon to provide the nurturing necessary to propel a student to higher cognitive levels. Although a few excellent public and private schools exist throughout the country at the elementary and secondary levels, even these do not always provide optimum conditions for their students. And, even if they could be counted on, there are too few such institutions and too many students in need of a great deal of enrichment.

So, as we've said, providing sufficient intellectual stimulation must ultimately fall to the parents or enrichment tutors of one kind or another who will be provided by the parents. Recall, the brain is like a muscle. It must be exercised or it will atrophy. The most effective brain "exercise" comes from a steady, low pressure, benign provision of various kinds of stimulation on a one-to-one basis. Again, *positive*

time spent in interesting but low-pressure cognitive training activities is the
most important gift a parent can give her child.

Parents today, faced with their working time and home time
stretched to the limits, might recoil from any suggestion that they
spend more time with their children or spend more time doing
much of anything except make a living and rest up in order to go
back to work again. I understand this and do not expect more than
can reasonably be given by any parent. However, parents should
endeavor to creatively involve other family members such as uncles,
aunts and especially grandparents in their child's life whenever
possible.

One way many of today's parents cover the childcare situation is
to provide a baby-sitter or childcare person on a daily basis. In Los
Angeles and in many other cities, the "nanny" of the past has been
supplanted by a housekeeper. These modern nannies often spend
more time with the child during the day than the parents do. They
may offer good, loving care. But, they probably don't provide high
quality language stimulation and other forms of cognitive stimulation. Kathleen Rogers, writing a community essay for the Los Angeles
Times regarding child care, states:

> The parents of these children (who are cared for by non-English speak-
> ing individuals) are vocal in their belief that it is a great advantage, that
> their children will grow up to be bilingual, when many of them already
> seem to me to be lagging in learning proper English.
>   Is multi-culturalism the goals of these parents, or is it really to save a
> little money on baby-sitting? Parents who have a choice should wake up
> and make the necessary sacrifices to invest in their children, who rep-
> resent America's future.[3]

We digressed here because the problem of the schools and the
problem of the parents is the same, the provision of high quality cognitive stimulation to children. However, both institutions seem to be
walking around the problem rather than dealing with it. Let's go back
to our discussion of the schools.

The mid-1960s marks the beginning of a decline in educational
standards and the "dumbing down" of education still continues today. Psychologists Richard Herrnstein and Charles Murray note that,
"One of the chief effects of the educational reforms of the 1960s was to
dumb down elementary and secondary education as a whole, making just about everything easier for the average student and easing
the demands on the gifted student....the dumbing down of text-
books permeated the textbook market, as publishers and authors

strove to satisfy school boards, which routinely applied 'readability' formulas to the books they were considering."[4]

Additionally, and perhaps looming larger than any other single factor in terms of the problems of educating our young people, has been the advent of television. At some point in the 1960s, television supplanted the printed page as the prime medium for receiving news, for recreation, and for shaping our ways of being and thinking. Television pacifies and titillates. It is enjoyable, but it does not offer much intellectual sustenance. It is passive, not interactive. The mind of the TV viewing child simply absorbs. What does this mind absorb? Basically, an awful melange of pap and nonsense with images changing at a rate of something like 2.3 per second! An advertisement appears approximately every three minutes of program time. Short attention spans have become the norm.

Our new national fad diagnosis is Attention Deficit Disorder (ADD). Can the decline in reading and writing skills, the rise in attention problems, the lack of focus, the sense of unrest and "dis-ease" (conditioned by ads which constantly exhort us to want something, buy something, go somewhere) be just *coincidental* with the devotion to watching television? It would hardly seem so.

Neil Postman, professor of communication arts and sciences at New York University, notes that television has "…by its power to control the time, attention and cognitive habits of our youth gained the power to control their education."[5] Postman goes on to say that, "Since our students will have watched approximately sixteen thousand hours of television by high school's end, questions should have arisen, even in the minds of officials at the Department of Education, about who will teach our students how to look at television, and when not to, and with what critical equipment when they do."

But, what's to be done? Television's power or influence is not losing its grip. Children read less and they often read only what a teacher assigns. Few children of my acquaintance read for pleasure. Few parents read to their children on a regular basis, though this would probably be the single best thing they could do in terms of enrichment. Many children today cannot focus on one train of thought for any length of time. We and our children are bombarded by stimuli from the TV set which we cannot, will not, or don't want to control.

To read a book requires some effort. One has to remember what has been read then sift and sort through ideas and create images from words. We move through the ideas in the book in a linear, logical manner. By contrast, TV requires nothing like this. TV comes at us in a sight and sound assault, dazzling us, mesmerizing us and dumbing us down.

It may be that computers and video games will lead us down a more productive intellectual path. Computer technology has potential. CD-Roms can be and often are highly imaginative and interactive. The interactivity is what sets the CD-Roms apart from the more passive world of television.

Actually, it is not difficult to imagine a CD-Rom "Gunfighter Gus" game, for example, with a protagonist who roams extensively through time and place in the Old West, teaching the history of the cattle drives, the treatment of native Americans, the trails through the Rockies and the Sierras and the gold strikes in California. The future of this technology's use to help maximize a child's intelligence is not clear yet, though the potential would appear to be considerable.

Whether schools will ever possess the resources to offer each child her own computer CD-Rom equipped or not does not seem likely at this point in time, given the financial difficulties of most school districts. Unfortunately, local, state and federal governments seem unable to contribute in any significant way to bring this high-tech component to schools in sufficient numbers to make a difference. Even when schools do have an adequate supply of computers, the length of time provided for learning computer skills is simply not enough. The standard forty-five or fifty-minute computer classes offered do not provide sufficient time to enable the student to explore the resources of the computer, become familiar with how to use programs, access on-line help, explore the internet, and generally, just spend time "fooling with" this technology.

Schools are an easy whipping boy these days. And I am not trying to add to their burdens. Most teachers in most schools are doing the best they can. However, all students—including the average and the very bright—are often shortchanged these days. Even if your child is of above-average intelligence, the question of whether or not he is receiving sufficient educational and intellectual stimulation from his school could legitimately be raised.

If education is being "dumbed down," if there are too many students and too many needs and too few teachers, if parents are often both working and surely very tired most evenings, will our children's intellectual levels simply drift downward or, at the least, not be maximized? Or are there other answers? In so many areas, it takes an adult human to teach a human child how to become fully human. Even if there was a computer for every child, many important areas of thought could not be adequately taught. It would appear difficult for a computer, for example, to help a child develop what James Wilson, Professor of Social Policy at UCLA, calls a "moral sense."[6] If most of us who have children or interface with children in some kind of teaching role find that we are dealing with too little time and/or too many children, where will we find more humanpower? Chapter 15 will talk about the problem of how to find more people to mentor and tutor our children.

NOTES

1. Ornstein, Allen and Levine, Daniel. *Foundations of Education, 4th Edition.* Boston: Houghton Mifflin. 1989. p. 156.
2. Ornstein and Levine, op cit p. 182.
3. Rogers, Kathleen. "A Real Nanny Dilemma," *Los Angeles Times* March 6, 1995.
4. Herrnstein, Richard & Murray, Charles. *The Bell Curve: intelligence and class structure in American life.* New York: Free Press. 1994. p. 430.
5. Postman, Neil. *Amusing Ourselves To Death.* New York: Viking. 1985. p. 145.
6. Wilson, James. *The Moral Sense.* New York: Free Press. 1993.

5

The Development of Intelligence: Environment is Decisive

Nature and nurture, genetic makeup and environment, both play major roles in determining an individual's intelligence level. We do not control who mates with whom as animal breeders do. Selective breeding is not desirable in our society. Thus, the hereditary aspect of intelligence is largely uncontrolled except that people with similar traits tend to mate and produce offspring often resembling themselves. For instance, two highly intelligent individuals who are interested in intellectual and cultural pursuits are more likely to meet and be interested in one another, perhaps ultimately producing children together, than is either one of these individuals likely to be romantically inclined toward an uneducated and unintelligent person. Social class too plays some part (often a large part) in determining whom we meet and marry. Social class may play a weaker role in the future, however. It appears that we are heading toward a society in which there will be a propensity for intelligent, well-educated people to work together, hang out together and marry and mate together. Such people are increasingly becoming the "cognitive elite" of our society.

Unless we are the rare individual disposed to selecting a mate principally for breeding purposes as in the case of a former professional athlete who stated that he chose a particular woman to be his wife because of her physical attributes which, when combined with his genetic endowments, would be likely to produce a star-athlete son many of us simply fall in love (or lust), get married, and have one or more babies.

All this is to say that most children's genetic intellectual makeup is derived mostly by chance, not by plan. Our children come into this world endowed with certain innate potentials in many different areas, including the area of the intelligences. Once they are conceived, practically speaking, there can be no altering of the genetic plan. The only alteration in the potentials of the human being is, as we've stated, through environmental interventions. Genetically, you are who you are; environmentally, you are who you might become. The environmental influence then, is laid, down over the genetic base structure. If the environment does not offer appropriate or sufficient nourishment or enrichment, the genetic endowment will not be able to blossom, no matter how good the genetic stock. In this regard, consider the following story of the Wild Boy of Aveyron:

> Lest anyone doubt that the environment matters in the development of intelligence, consider the rare and bizarre cases in which a child is hidden away in a locked room by a demented adult or breaks free of human contact altogether and runs wild...we know that if the isolation from human society lasts for years, rather than for just months, the children are intellectually stunted for life. Such was...the experience of the "Wild Boy of Aveyron," discovered in southern France soon after the Revolution and the establishment of the first French Republic....
>
> The 12- or 13-year old boy had been found running naked in the woods, mute, wild, and evidently out of contact with humanity for most of his life...as it turned out, neither he, nor the others like him that we know about, resemble Rousseau's noble savage in the least. Most of them never learn to speak properly or become independent adults...They seem unable to become fully human despite the heroic efforts to restore them to society. From these rare cases we can draw a hopeful conclusion: *If the ordinary human environment is so essential for bestowing human intelligence, we should be able to create extraordinary environments to raise it further.* (italics added)[1]

Two highly intelligent individuals who have children together will not likely see their child exceed themselves in terms of IQ. Two people who are very limited intellectually—perhaps borderline retarded in IQ—will not likely have children with lower intelligence than they, but rather, of higher intelligence. This is because of the "regression to the mean" effect, which tends to pull in the "tails" of a distribution in this case the distribution of IQ over time.[2] From an evolutionary standpoint, this particular effect has probably kept the human population in a more or less safe, middle-of-the road course in the distribution of intelligence, as well as many other factors such as height, strength, health, weight, speed, and so on.

The heritability of intelligence is generally considered to be forty percent to sixty percent. If we say that fifty percent is a good approximation regarding the inheritance factor, this obviously leaves fifty percent for the environmental factor in the nature-nurture equation. This means that each of us has about half of our potential at birth. Clearly, whether our environments are rich or poor in terms of intellectual stimulation makes a very large difference.

How do we enrich an environment? What happens when we do? As previously discussed, experiments with laboratory mice concluded that an enriched environment (defined as more things to crawl on, around, under; more things to see and hear) increases the weight of the brain, even in older animals.[3] Researcher Dr. Ruth Winter noted that the brains of the young mice from the enriched environments were not only heavier, but also more chemically active. This indicated rich interconnections among brain cells and greater metabolic activity than those of litter mates living alone in an "impoverished" environment. We enrich the environment of the human child in much the same way we do for a mouse, by providing many things to look at, talk to, hear, touch, and smell. In most homes, the normal environment could be considered one of at least average or "good enough" enrichment. However, since we are looking to enhance intellectual potential, we would want to be sure to provide above-average stimulation.

The crib and playroom should contain many interesting things to look at, hear and touch. Television is not an enriching factor. It is too passive, and its sounds and pictures are not connected to anything the child can relate to. A learning organism such as a child needs high interactivity and needs to have a response to her behaviors. In other words, she needs to interact with the environment rather than be just a passive observer. When she smiles, someone should be there to smile back—otherwise, the child's smiles become less frequent. When she gurgles or coos and makes various sounds, she needs another person to respond in kind. This type of interactivity is very important for intellectual development.

The creation of a good or enriched physical environment is the easy part. Add music, lots of talk, and provide things to touch. Include peek-a-boo faces and smiles; be gentle and lovingly pick up and hold the child. This is the start of a very good environment.

To this physical environment, add other people and your adult speech. We suggest that the parent drop into a form of talk called "motherese" or "caretaker speech." Caretaker speech, according to clinicians who work with infants and very young children, "...facilitates language acquisition because it intuitively utilizes patterns and sounds consistent with the child's developing linguistic abilities. Far from 'talking down' to children, caretaker speech reflects a remarkable unconscious knowledge of the structure of language and the nature of the process of language acquisition. Thus, with some very simple techniques...adults [can] manage to facilitate [the child's] understanding, communication, and the incredibly complex process of language acquisition..."[4]

An enriched environment for the infant involves being surrounded by language spoken from a real person, not language from TV or video (though these would probably be better than nothing). One afternoon, I overheard the following exchange by a "super mom" in a market.

> Shall we get this triangle tip for daddy's dinner tonight? You know, he just loves this dish. We'll also cook up mashed potatoes and some green beans. Umm, good! Now, what do we need for dessert? Some ice cream, maybe. Come on. Let's go over to the ice cream freezer and we'll pick up some of that cherry flavor that dad likes so much. You are such a good shopper, a big help to mom.

And so on. Far from being bored, the child fixed his eyes on his mother's face, occasionally looking to see where she was pointing, evidently riveted on the flow of rich language inflections emanating from his mother's mouth. Her tone was pleasant and conversational. If her baby made a sound, she considered it an affirmative reply of some sort. Her language was highly interactive with the child's sounds and gazes.

The mother's language assists the child in developing his own language skills, though in general, speech *per se* cannot be hurried. Children understand and use words before they can speak words. Let speech and language develop within a matrix of meaningful, soft, loving talk from the parent to the child, between parents and between parents and others. Although the child may not yet be able to talk, he can listen and observe.

One of the very important basic skills a child begins to develop in early childhood is responding appropriately to a number of different verbal stimuli. It is important for the child's developing intelligence that he learn to focus on relevant items in his environment. The child should respond well to instructions such as "Watch what I do," or "This is the way it goes" or "Be careful on the stairs" and so on. If the child does not learn to pay good attention to the words and warnings of others, he will not be as effective in his environment, whether this be at home, grandmother's house, preschool, or playing at a park with other children.

Although the concept of more toys and playthings appears to be a good one for mice, it takes all these things plus interactive language to begin to move the child toward his fullest cognitive potentials. A kind adult who will talk to and with the child is the key. Keep in mind that the adult should not just fill the air with a lot of word-gibberish. This does not constitute an enrichment program. The adult should use her already well-developed language skills to pair objects with words (Here is a book, This is a spoon, Do you want some Cheerios?) and to teach the child to attend as stated above.

Incredibly, it appears that "love" may be learned, too. And, certainly, how to be "loving" and capable of eliciting positive responses from others is a very important skill for any child to learn. This and much more is learned as the child grows up. Whatever is learned can be taught. It is up to the adult to figure out what is worth teaching and how to go about instructing her child. This might seem an imposing task for most parents unless they are child development specialists. To assist parents in the overall training of their child up to the kindergarten level, we will rely on an adaptation of an instrument known as the Behavioral Analysis Rating Instrument, or as we will refer to it fondly from now on, the BARI.

The BARI offers parents a way to know where their preschool child stands on the developmental ladder and what specific set of behaviors might deserve attention for development. Children who are competent on the higher levels of the BARI will be ready for kindergarten in almost any school. The complete BARI program will be found in Part II of this book. This program has been been shown to be effective. You can use all or any part(s) of the BARI training program, and as you will see, much latitude is given to parents who want to individualize any and all training for their child. From a BARI perspective, this is fine because the focus of the program is to teach to a level of competency, not necessarily instruct by any specific method.

Since the BARI will take us approximately up to age five, we will turn our attention now to assisting development through ages five or six to ten or so. Part III will focus on the concepts of "domains of intelligence" and the "building blocks" of thinking skills.

NOTES

1. Herrnstein, Richard and Murray, Charles. *The Bell Curve*. New York: Free Press. 1994. p. 410.
2. Wallis, W. Allen and Roberts, Harry. *Statistics: a new approach*. Glencoe: Free Press, 1956. p. 258.
3. Winter, Ruth. "Biomarkers: beating body burnout," *American Health*, May, 1984, pp. 70-80.
4. Donovan, Denis and McIntyre, Deborah. *Healing the Hurt Child*. New York: Norton, 1990. p. 13.

6

Getting Started

At this point, let's assume you are convinced that most parents, yourself included, don't work as effectively as they might to enhance their child's cognitive potential. Also, let's say you've decided to embark on a cognitive enhancement program as suggested in this book. In short, you feel as I do that most children have untapped intellectual potential and that such potential can be enhanced by certain easy and pleasant everyday activities. Other than reading the rest of this book, how do you start?

Let's start with an example, an all too common one, I fear—of a young parent who heard about cognitive coaching, then decided to work with his daughter, only to become immediately frustrated by her lack of response.

NEIL AND JENNY

Two-year old Jenny is the apple of Neil's eye. He loves her and dotes on her every smile and sound. Jenny is his first child, and he never felt he could love anyone so much.

When Neil heard about early cognitive stimulation or ways in which parents can maximize their child's cognitive skills, he immediately grasped the idea, decided that neither he nor Jenny's mother was providing sufficient stimulation to the child, and embarked on his own "homemade" program.

Neil knew, however, that just about every early childhood expert recommended cognitive development by reading to

39

the child. He had vaguely heard of some kind of
language called "motherese." Neil discussed providing more
language stimulation to Jenny with his wife, Becky, who was
agreeable to such a program, but basically felt that the
everyday environment she provided Jenny was sufficient. Neil
did not agree and decided to read more to Jenny,
and to try to cut down on TV and videotime for her.

Neil was quickly surprised to find that Jenny, after an initial few
pleasant moments in her daddy's arms with a book, was not
overly interested in being read to, and in fact, would quickly
station herself back in front of the TV set. Neil was somewhat
dismayed as well as a bit alarmed over Jenny's apparent
preference for TV or video programs.

Neil called an expert, his grandmother, for some advice on how to
deal with Jenny, books and TV. She advised "hooking"
Jenny to the book by talking in a much more animated voice, pointing
to pictures, making up part of the story if that would be more
interesting for Jenny, asking her questions as they went along
(motherese), keeping the "reading" sessions short, using books
with colorful and interesting pictures. Neil's grandmother also told
him to continue to cut down on the TV and videos for Jenny.

Jenny and Neil were soon enjoying their reading sessions together,
though the parents also had to curtail the amount of TV watching,
including the various children's videos they had. Rather quickly,
Jenny showed that she very much liked being read to, as she would
bring books to her parents and request what they had come to call
"book time."

When we, as parents, begin to attempt a cognitive enhancement
program of even the "mildest" and seemingly most pleasant sort,
such as board games like Candyland for the younger set or Monopoly
for older children, we are always competing with television. Television
is the true "Great Satan" from the standpoint of cognitive enhancement. Although there are programs which offer much in the way of
information, children rarely choose to watch such programs voluntarily.
And by definition, no television program is interactive. Once a child
has been introduced to TV and videos, other forms of stimulation
tend to pale in comparison. It is difficult for most of us or many other
activities to be as entertaining as TV.

Learning should be enjoyable, even though it is not always easy.
Learning and becoming more competent in many areas is rewarding
for most children. From competency comes confidence and positive

self-esteem. However, if your child has become "television and video conditioned," it can be much more difficult to entice him into "slow-speed" activities such as listening to stories, playing board games, coloring or reading.

Jenny, in the above example, had been exposed to television and video programs for most of her life. If we estimate that she had watched video or children's TV programs for 3 hours per day since she was a year old, in that twelve-month period Jenny would have spent some 1,095 hours, or 45.6 days of her very young life, in front of the TV set. That's twelve percent of her second year and about six percent of her entire life! If she watched 5 hours per day on average she would have spent 1,825 hours or some 76 days in front of TV since her first birthday or twenty one percent of her life since that time in front of TV. As we all know, some children spend many more hours than 3 or 5 per day viewing TV or videos. In some homes the TV is on almost 100 percent of the time. It's a great babysitter but a lousy cognitive enhancer.

Jenny, like many children, had been trained on TV, conditioned for the experience, as it were. She enjoyed, of course, the sound and color and stimulation provided by the various children's videos available, or even the insipid cartoons offered on some channels. Jenny had learned the songs from videos. She moved to the rhythms. Her face lit up when she recognized a familiar melody. Although it is delightful to observe her responses, Jenny has been deprived in important ways. She does not interact or problem-solve with this medium. She does not develop the foundation to use her own imagination when older. She does not practice basic thinking skills which involve cause-effect sequencing in linear fashion (for example, we turn the page; we pause the story; we place the toys just so). She does not learn how to delay gratification, to pause a bit, to enjoy a slower pace. Instead, Jenny is bombarded by sounds and images which flit across the screen and into her brain in a rapid, ever-changing fashion.

If you are going to start a cognitive enhancement program with a child who has been pre-conditioned to television, be prepared for some necessary creative activity on your part. Initially, the amount of TV watching time needs to be reduced. You must set up "quiet times" when there is little going on in the child's environment except what she causes to happen. For example, encourage the little one to play with her toys or books, play outside or bang on pots with a spoon. The older children can have the option of participating in quiet activities such as puzzles, board games, reading, or play in the yard. These activities not only help wean the child from TV, but they aid in the development of imagination and creativity. The quiet time allows you, the parent, to introduce various activities of your own choosing which set the stage for cognitive enhancement, as well as promote a positive bond between you and your child.

Looked at in another way, if the child has become so "television-dependent" that whatever you propose is boring, then gradually cut back TV time and substitute the more enriching activities slowly. Do *not* make the mistake of turning off the TV and saying something to the effect that there will be more reading or talking or whatever now that the TV is off. In other words, don't link the reduction in TV with your cognitive stimulation program. Reduce TV first, allow the child to do her own activities or those you propose or even to do nothing. After a suitable time has passed and this could be from a few days to a few weeks then introduce your own brand of fun as part of your cognitive enrichment program. It would be tantamount to the *Cat In the Hat* character showing up on a boring, rainy day when, some afternoon, you indicate that you have a great idea called coloring with crayons, making pictures with chalk on a cement patio (with washable chalk, of course), Chutes and Ladders, or card games such as War or Crazy Eights, or other games such as Trivial Pursuit for Children, Othello, chess or checkers.

We're not advocating that there be no TV in your family's life. However, we are recommending cautious and sensible use of TV. It is understandable that parents use the TV set as a kind of hypnotic device to help keep the kids quiet while dinner is being prepared and so on. However, if you do use it in this way, you may be depriving your child of a chance to develop her own imagination and stretch her intelligence, not to mention her independence from the stimulation of TV. In many families, TV is used as a kind of generalized background noise, like the fire in a hearth in olden days. Once your family becomes accustomed to this mindless murmuring, it may be difficult to wean the children or the adults from it.

Before TV (yes, there was such a time), children managed to wait for dinner without being entertained. Or, rather, they entertained themselves by playing with toys, reading comic books, playing ball outside, resting and thinking, and so on. Why do so many parents seem to feel that their children must be provided unending and constant pleasurable stimulation? Actually, most of us would be happy if such pleasurable stimulation came from a picture or story book. Children who read for pleasure seem to be "winners" in all sorts of academic and other situations. The same surely cannot be said for television. If TV watching produced more brain power, our knowledge base would be exploding by now. If TV enhanced intellectual and academic performance, the SAT scores of our college-bound young people would not have shown an almost continuous decline over the past few decades, nor would the achievement scores in most of our key big city school districts be so low.

You do your child a favor when you reduce TV viewing time and, of course, the various videos which are part of children's TV fare. The Disney videos and other videos for children are terrific, no doubt about it. But they should not be the backbone of our children's intellectual development. It is one thing to view the seven dwarfs and Snow White on screen—it is another kind of experience entirely to read or hear this story read.

Bruno Bettelheim has illuminated the enormous help fairy tales can be as the child wrestles with growing up and becoming a person.[1] The fairy tale which we read to the child or which he reads to himself, as well as many other types of stories, enhance the emotional realms of the child's development while also expanding the cognitive realms. The child must think, consider, perceive cause and effect, digest the implications of the story, and incorporate story elements into his own growing-up difficulties. Although a particular video may have a story-line which is thought provoking, the video by its nature moves quickly. This makes it impossible for the child to stop at some point in the story to pause and reflect.

Videos, when shown over and over, become as dulling as a story read on a tape again and again. In both instances, the story line, the words and thoughts lose effectivenss as consciousness and cognitive expanders because they don't have the flexibility and creativity of a parent's voice. Rather, videos become simply part of the background noise within a household. Nothing special. But a story told by an adult, full of voice inflections and facial cues, can be something very special for the young listener. When a mother tells the child about the witch who *swooped* down from the black sky above and observes his excited face, she should then file this word and scene away in her memory for possible use in another story, another surprise for the child. The parent has control of the thematic material and the drama she adds can stimulate the imagination of the child. By doing this she expands his cognitive and creative grasp. Even if the expansion seems ever so slight, it is there and it is real.

Let's talk for a moment about how to talk to the young child as opposed to the four and five year olds and up. As mentioned earlier, "motherese" is effective with infants and very young children, probably up to age two or three, depending on the child. Motherese, or caretaker talk, does not come naturally to all adults, but for those who can use it, communication with the child is enhanced. Child psychologists, Denis Donovan and Deborah McIntyre, note:

> Caretaker speech facilitates language acquisition because it intuitively utilizes patterns and sounds consistent with the child's developing linguistic abilities. Far from 'talking down' to children, caretaker speech reflects a remarkable unconscious knowledge of the structure of the process of language acquisition.[2]

The linguist, B.A. Moskowitz, explains, "Caretaker speech is a distinct speech register that differs from others in its simplified vocabulary, the systematic phonological simplifications of some words, higher pitch, exaggerated intonation, short, simple sentences and a high proportion of questions (among mothers) or imperatives (among fathers)."[3] Infants are responsive to caretaker speech or motherese even when the adult is using a language different from that used by the baby's parents. It appears to be a case of not what you say but how you say it.

This brings us back to Neil and countless parents like him (not just fathers). Until he put some life into his voice, Jenny was not absorbed in what he was reading to her, even though the book, according to Neil, was "...an award winner with great pictures." When Neil pumped energy and vitality into his voice and pointed to the pictures, the whole book came alive and Jenny began to enjoy the experience. Incidentally, Jenny is now an avid book-looker and a good story listener now. Neil is an enthusiastic and imaginative reader. The bond created between parent and child through reading leads toward the child becoming a lifelong lover of books.

In addition to developing your story-telling, story-reading and conversational skills with your child, you need to place somewhere on your walls or in your mind the slogan DO NOT PRESSURE THIS CHILD. Also, if what you talk about and do with your child, including reading, is not easy and interesting for both you and the child then you probably should not do it since you will only tend to turn the child off to such learning interactions with you and, possibly, with books and teachers altogether. If Neil was not able to generate enough interest in the book he was reading to Jenny to hold her attention, then better to drop the activity. Follow the child's lead, with the exception of TV, do something that interests her while gradually stimulating interest in other things you would like to see her do.

ARE WE HAVING FUN YET?

Let's say your child is playing somewhat randomly with her dolls and other toys one afternoon. If this is a time you have set aside for cognitive enrichment, it would probably be a mistake to *insist* that she read a book with you instead, though you might offer her this option. A probably more productive move on your part would be to sit on the floor near her without intruding or taking over her play. Initially, however, you, too, might engage in some basic doll play, or find interesting things to do with other manipulable toys.

If one of your goals has been to practice fine-motor coordination, then you and the child can gradually play with the toys or crayons which provide such practice. You can pick up blocks and build simple towers or bridges or string beads, for instance. This may last only for a few minutes before the young child tires of the activity. You may continue what you are doing for a bit until you realize that the child is really not likely to return to that activity in the next few minutes. If the child has, instead, begun leafing through a picture book, you might do the same with another book, taking care not to grab the child's book out of her hands. You should not intrude on or take over every activity the child initiates. If you do, she soon won't initiate much of anything. So, add to but don't insist on the child's enjoyment with a particular activity.

There is an art to playing with children when you are using a cognitive enrichment program. You must introduce language and ideas and guide without pressuring. You need to expand the child's world and develop creativity through play and stories, yet not have the child become dependent on you for his play activities. Thus, sometimes there is "playing together" while at other times the child will require clear signals from you that it is time for him to play alone. Ambivalence in this matter on the part of the parent leads to confusion and unhappiness on the part of the child.

With an older child, staying with an activity is often easier once you have decided on a mutually enjoyable game such as checkers or cards. After age four or five (see discussion of the "five to seven shift" in chapter 12) you should avoid the use of motherese and move toward "Hemingwayese." In other words, use short, simple sentences which are clear and to the point. No long, convoluted Faulkner-style sentences here. Just speak plainly about whatever you want to talk about. It is best to avoid always being the Question Asker, though some demonstration of interest in the child's life is, of course, always appropriate. It is good practice to respect the child's developing conversational abilities, while speaking simply. Avoid talking down. Talk about things that you have done or topics that interest you.

Children learn through positive interactions with older, interesting tutors. Most parents are good teachers though sometimes they become less interesting to the child because they are pushing too hard. Added to this situation though is the reality of the fact that we are the parent and the child is our child. We can be friendly, but we are not really friends. We provide structure and guidance and have to say the "no's" which may create resentment. But, if we are pretty good parents, we will have a lot of credits in the child's emotional bank. Thus, he will be able to differentiate between times when we are his chess playing pal and times when we have to remind him to turn out the light because it's bedtime.

To summarize. To get started on a program of maximizing your child's cognitive development there are several points to keep in mind.

1. Reduce your child's television watching time by turning off the set and setting up "quiet time." During quiet time, allow no one in the family, including parents, to watch TV.

2. Develop an interesting repertoire or "patter" of your own. If you are presenting material in a dull way, why would the child be interested?

3. Don't force the child to engage in some enrichment activity he does not like or does not want to do at that time.

You can't create a liking for something by using pressure. You create a liking for or love of learning things by your own learning and by engaging the child in age-appropriate activities that are enjoyable and in appropriate time bits. Insisting that the child sit still and learn four opening chess moves before you let him go to bed for the night will probably cause him to develop a negative attitude toward both chess and you.

The message here is, "Stimulate the child's mind without hurting his feelings." Or, plant the seeds without stomping the ground too much. Learn to observe your child. Start where her interests are, not where yours are. A good tutor or coach can virtually start anywhere and teach anything. So, before you get started, think about your child and what kind of person he is, what he likes or does not like to do.

Think about the thinking process, about intelligence and what it is. If the child is under age five, go through some of the various items presented in the next few chapters. Where does your child fit in on these little developmental segments? If your child is between five and ten, skim through Part III and see where she may need some help in further development, or just take a look at areas that might interest you to do with your child.

It is best to take a slow, easy, steady approach to assist a child's cognitive development. A crash program is inadvisable and won't work. Just assume that helping your child learn how to think effectively is a big part of your job as a parent. Fortunately it is an interesting and rewarding task.

NOTES

1. Bettelheim, Bruno. *The Uses of Enchantment: the meaning and importance of fairy tales.* New York: Knopf. 1976.
2. Donovan, Denis and McIntyre, Deborah. *Healing the Hurt Child.* New York: Norton. 1990. p. 13.
3. Moskowitz, B.A. "The Acquisition of Language," *Scientific American,* November, 1978.

II

THE FIRST FIVE YEARS

7

Starting the BARI Program

Once a baby is conceived and begins to grow, the learning process starts. The baby continues to learn rapidly after birth and then, of course, throughout all stages of life. The human being, from start to finish, is probably the most efficient and omnivorous learning machine ever to grace the earth. As the shark has evolved to hunt and eat, the human has evolved to learn.

As stated previously, the learning that takes place in the first few years of life is generally considered to be the most important learning of all. This early learning is the foundation for the intellect which will gradually form during the remainder of the child's first decade of life, those ten crucial years that will set the stage for most of what we can or cannot become in later life.

Intelligence is not, as many assume, simply book smarts. It includes but is not limited to being able to correctly answer many Jeopardy show questions and get good grades in school. Being able to think logically, perceive the consequences of one's actions, think vicariously, remember well, and express oneself well in speech or writing involves a highly important form of intelligence—*verbal intelligence*. It is largely our verbal intelligences that enable us to read, write, and discuss ideas well. It may be the most important of the intelligences for academic success. Even so, it is only one of several important forms of intelligence.

Quantitative intelligence or facility with math and computers may, in the future, come to be more valued than verbal intelligence. And both verbal and mathematical intelligences may in many instances be less important than *social intelligence*. The latter represents one's ability to creatively grapple with the many aspects and demands of daily life in a crowded and complex world.

51

Intellect in its broadest sense stands for the myriad of things which humans learn to do ranging across various realms of dance, art, music, the abstractions of math and physics, athletics, drama, philosophy, building, planning, politics and so on. Intellect also encompasses the learning and use of the subtle social skills so important in jobs such as psychotherapy, teaching, sales, and political positions in democratic governments.

Possessing one of the intelligences to a high degree does not preclude possessing other cognitive skills. A highly verbal attorney or professor might, for example, also be a gifted woodworker, musician or athlete. We have our various talents and some of our talents are in greater demand in our society than are others. For the Eskimo, a highly developed intelligence involves an acutely sensitive spatial orientation. This spatial orientation sense is necessary for one who must move about among large expanses in drifts of snow without street signs to point the way. Although a good sense of spatial orientation might be useful in some circumstances in our society, it is perhaps not as important as other intellectual skills might be.

A parent in our society would be confident if her child developed strong language, math and social skills. She would probably not be concerned with the thought that her child may not be able to find his way home in the unlikely event (in our society) of a blinding snowstorm. An Eskimo mother, of course, would probably take an entirely different view.

Every child needs to possess a reasonably well-developed cluster of the basic intellectual skills necessary for survival in his environment. In our high-tech society, skills involving language, math, computer, monetary exchange, and social interaction are highly useful. Skills involving hunting, fishing, running, jumping, swimming, use of a compass, gathering berries, hitting a ball, or discerning ocean currents may not be as critically useful as the first grouping for sheer survival, though they may add much to the quality of life.

THE TASK OF PARENTS

It seems safe to say that most parents today are rightly convinced that the acquisition of good basic thinking skills is very important for their child. Parents tend to be highly aware of the intellectual and social development of their children. The current generation of parents may be better informed in this area than any previous one. Today's parents tend to be goal-oriented and desirous of the "best" they can acquire for their child. Together with love, care, and nurturance, a principal task of the modern parent is to prepare her child for life outside the home environment and for what has become the first stage of formal education, kindergarten.

In order to accomplish this goal, the parent must give careful consideration to the child's development in four major areas:

- Physical-Coordinative
- Language-Cognitive
- Aesthetic-Creative
- Social-Emotional

All of these areas involve forms of intelligence. Combined, they maximize the child's various intellectual propensities and lay the groundwork for further development in the second half of the child's first ten years as we'll discuss in Part III.

The physical-coordinative area involves large and small muscle coordination. Language-cognitive functioning involves skills such as recognition of shapes, numbers, expressive and receptive language, memory and rudimentary cause-effect thinking. The aesthetic-creative domain has to do with music, arts and crafts and the enjoyment and understanding of the physical world. The social-emotional domain of intelligence involves skills in dealing with peers, response to separation or new situations and the budding awareness of self and others.

THE STRUCTURE OF THE PROGRAM

The basic premises of this program are the following:

1. Parents desire and would respond favorably to a planned and well thought out but informal and non-pressuring program by which they could more systematically and effectively assist their child's development in the four key areas

2. Parents want to be aware early of any developmental lags their child may experience in any of the four areas

3. Parents desire information about what steps to take to address any such developmental lags with appropriate teaching procedures and

4. Parents desire that their child be "kindergarten ready" at approximately five years of age. This is because kindergarten is the first stage of the formal learning process for children in our society and thus an important academic/intellectual starting point.

The Behavioral Analysis Rating Instrument (BARI) was developed by the author to promote and enhance a child's development.[1] The BARI consists of many items which have to do with the child's developmental status in the various major areas noted above. The BARI is both diagnostic and prescriptive. Preschools which use the BARI do new ratings every three to six months on each child. This is to keep fresh in the teacher's mind the needs of each individual child. It is also to chart the developmental course of each child. As the child develops and becomes more competent in various areas, his "scores" rise, as they should. All of this will be further clarified in the discussion below.

Use of the BARI begins with the parent initially checking the items corresponding to what the child can or cannot yet do in various areas. Then, the parent merely begins a simple program of *teaching to the next level up on each item*. The assessment is informal and does *not* involve testing the child. A sample item involving cooperation is shown below. Since it is expected that the child's development will be evaluated more than once over a period of time, usually every six months, most parents find it helpful to date the time of their rating. Again, please recall that the child is *not* tested; rather, the parent simply circles the items that best describe her child.

Cooperation with peers (circle one)

Date of 1st rating _____ 2nd rating _____ 3rd rating _____

1. Cannot or will not.

2. Unwillingly cooperates and only with much adult guidance.

3. Cooperates reluctantly, but will do so with adult encouragement.

4. Generally cooperates willingly, though may need some adult prompting.

5. Almost always cooperates well with other children.

Let's say that you checked your child's cooperative behavior with peers as being at about the 2 level. The simple task, then, is to help your child attain the 3 level, then the 4 level and so on. Under each rating box in the chapters to come will be suggestions for activities which will help the child acquire the desired skill. These are by no means all the activities which could be used and parents will be able to think of others well-suited to their own individual child and circumstances.

After the initial rating, the parent begins a gentle teaching program which is informal and individualized. This teaching program utilizes pleasant activities that will engage the child. When the parent is able to circle all 4s or 5s, the child is "kindergarten ready" from an intellectual/developmental standpoint. At this point, the parent will have taken the initial major steps toward maximizing her child's cognitive skills.

This program is not complicated. It is easy to follow and quite straightforward. You will also perceive how easy it is for you to be alert to opportunities to informally advance your child's development in many ways. It is very important, however, that you realize that the BARI program is neither a "test" as in school nor a structured preplanned teaching program.

Let's take another practice example. Item 1 of the BARI asks for your assessment of your child's overall body movement. Obviously, the answer will reflect your opinion but each number provides some idea of the way your child should look in order for you to circle a particular number. The young child will, naturally, be very unsure of himself or, perhaps, you will choose "slow and clumsy" and circle number 2. You simply circle the item which best reflects your honest assessment of the child's ability on this item having to do with Overall Body Movement.

This will be the case on every BARI item. You may rate them all at once, or when you are moved to do so. Each item is developmentally based. A "low" number for the younger child is expected, while the more skilled, older child will be rated higher. Low scores are not inherently "bad," they reflect only the status of the child's skill level on the item being rated.

Item 1. Overall Body Movement (circle one)

Date of 1st rating _____ 2nd rating _____ 3rd rating _____

1. Very unsure of self.

2. Slow and clumsy; movements are awkward.

3. Fairly sure of body movements.

4. Sure of body movements; smooth and well-integrated movements most of the time.

5. Completely at ease with movement of body; good balance and coordination.

As stated, all you do is circle the number of the description *which best describes your child*. Remember, please, that your rating should reflect only what your child is truly doing, not what you think he could do or feel that he might do soon. To benefit you and your child, your ratings on every item must be absolutely honest and based only on what you have observed. When in doubt, score low.

What is the purpose of all this, you ask, other than to raise parental anxiety when you see that your child is not yet getting all 5s circled (this usually will not happen until the child is a late four year old or early five year old). There are two primary purposes to the ratings:

1. To assess your child's developmental status in the area rated and then to develop, if you so desire, an informal teaching program to help him in that area and,

2. To act as a guide to assist you in what level you need to teach to in order to move the child along developmentally.

Beneath each of the BARI items there is a discussion of the nature of the item and suggestions for teaching toward the next higher level of competency until, by age four or five, the child is completely competent in the areas assessed. You needn't be bound by the suggestions, however. Try to "get the idea" of what is required, feel free to try any and everything which might interest you and your child as it seems to related to the item.

Above all, do *not* turn enjoyable time with your child into a pedantic, boring, and stressful "teaching time." These concepts have been derived from the fact that children are natural learners, that parents do a great deal of teaching, and that all the time spent may be more useful for the child's development if parents are following some reasonably structured program in a *reasonably unstructured* manner.

Initially, some parents have found the BARI to be intimidating because it *seemed* long and complicated. But it is neither. All you need do is study an item, think about your child, then circle his approximate skill level. Again, please do not set up a series of "tests" for your child to see how he "scores" on an item. If the child has not performed the behavior specified, then rate him a 1 in that area and start a gentle developmental program from that point.

Another purpose of the BARI ratings is diagnostic in nature. There are some children for whom the maturing process takes longer and these children may manifest mild developmental delays or maturational lags in one or more areas of the BARI ratings system. If a healthy, normal four or five year old is receiving honest ratings from you and perhaps your spouse of, say, 2s or 3s on some items, then he may be lagging a bit in those areas.

If you feel that your child may be lagging developmentally, do not panic and certainly do not take the BARI as the final diagnostic word. Consult with your spouse or some trusted family member, the child's preschool teacher and your pediatrician. Perhaps your observations are not accurate, or you misunderstood the item, or perhaps the child has a mild maturational delay. In this case, consultation with relevant and appropriate professionals may be needed.

To repeat. A preponderance of 4 and 5 ratings on all items indicates a kindergarten-ready child.

A few general considerations:

- Parents should consider each item in a broad sense. Don't be "picky" or too particular and fail to rate the item just because it may not be phrased as well as you would prefer. Your wording may be more appropriate to you than mine; we all have our own style.

- Be conservative. When in doubt rate low. This is no reflection on the child. Rating low is a safeguard.

- This is *not* an age-graded scale. You should rate on an absolute basis. That is, you either see the behavior or you don't. The child can either perform the item in the manner specified or he can't. Do not judge whether the behavior is being performed well or poorly "compared to most three year olds" but only whether it is being performed at all according to the item choices.

- Expect low scores from young ones. As the child becomes older, his scores will rise.

- Rate again every five or six months.

- Finally, each item includes many suggestions for ways in which parents can attempt to enhance development in that area. Use these activities or others which you deem more suitable and appropriate for you and your child.

NOTE

1.   Gardner, James. *Considerations: a guide for teachers and parents on the growth and development of preschool children.* Los Angeles: Wildwood 1974.

8

Physical Development

Sensorimotor development, including good small and large muscle coordination, is the basis for development of cognitive functioning as well as social skills, both of which eventually affect one's self-esteem. Although there have been individuals who were born without the ability to develop normal overall coordination yet still were able to achieve amazing things, the fact remains that, in general, higher cognitive and social skills rest on a base of good overall coordinative development.

The Discussion in Part II is less general and far more specific than the previous chapters. In this section and three subsequent sections, various behaviors of the child will be highlighted, followed by information about a range of skill levels which will range for most young children from "cannot do" to "can do very well." The skill-level range is to help us keep in mind that the child usually does not jump from being unable to do something to suddenly mastering the particular activity completely. We generally crawl before we walk and walk before we run. Following the range of skill levels for each item are comments as to why the skill is important, how you can blend it with other activities, and how you might best develop that skill for your child.

As you read the items, you will doubtless perceive that your child may need little or no help in some areas, while he may require a lot of help in others. Also, the suggestions for things to do are just that, suggestions. They are meant to point a way, not be the end-all in instruction. Once an interested parent gets the idea here, she may even add many more activities in more subtle and skillful ways than those mentioned in this book. Again, enjoy the book. Enjoy your child. Be easy with the child and with yourself.

GENERAL COORDINATION

Item 1. Overall Body Movement (circle one)

Date of 1st rating ——————— 2nd rating ——————— 3rd rating ———————

1. Very unsure of self.

2. Slow and clumsy; movements are awkward.

3. Fairly sure of body movements.

4. Sure of body movements; smooth and well-integrated most of the time.

5. Completely at ease with movement of body; good balance and coordination.

Almost any kind of activity involving whole body movement will facilitate the development of the child's coordination, sureness, grace and balance. In general, allow the child free play in interesting environments such as playgrounds with climbing or swinging equipment suitable for young children; hallways in the home where push or roll toys may be used; shallow swimming pools; and so on. MacDonald's Restaurants have some interesting playgrounds designed by child development specialists which are brightly colored and include bounce balls, doors, steps and slides. You can get many ideas of your own from just looking at a well-constructed play environment designed for young children.

Although most of us can't duplicate something like the local playground or a MacDonald's play area, we can still devise some very interesting play areas in our own homes or backyards. In England, one can find "junk playgrounds" constructed with surplus cargo nets, boxes and the like. Again, this may be a bit much for the average household, but you can use these ideas to generate some interesting places for your own children to roam. Tree houses, doll houses, water slides, forts, teeter-totters and swings are some examples of play-type constructions that may fit into your backyard.

These home playgrounds are not only fun and inspire adventure but, also, the child's peers become involved and add to the enjoyment. A slightly older child who has more dexterity on swings or slides or climbing toys can help a younger child overcome his timidity and add to the fun as well. If you are trying to encourage your child to use playground toys, it is usually best to allow your child to be exposed to other children who are already using and enjoying playground equipment. It is better for him to act more or less at his own pace than for you to strongly insist that he try the sliding board, jungle gym, diving board or whatever.

Item 2. Walking (circle one)

Date of 1st rating _____ 2nd rating _____ 3rd rating _____

1. Cannot walk at all.
2. Needs to cling to adults or to furniture.
3. Unsure and clumsy, often falls or sits, but walks independently.
4. Unsure and clumsy but does not fall too often and walks independently.
5. Stable and sure of self; walks without falling and entirely independently.

By age two or before, most children have crawled and some have walked. Initially, we help the child practice walking by offering our own hand for support and walking along with the child. A standing child can be encouraged to start walking from a stable point such as a table. He then can take steps toward the parent who positions herself close by so that the child initially need only take a few steps before reaching the comfort of the parent's arms. As the child becomes an increasingly skilled walker, the parent can move farther and farther away in the room. Encouraging this activity in a room with carpeting helps cushion falls early on, though a carpet that is overly plush and thick should be avoided since the child may have difficulty maintaining balance.

Following the development of basic walking, the parent may want to introduce activities such as Step on Squares or Step on Lines, for example. Drawn with washable chalk on cement almost any set of squares, triangles or lines can be utilized. This helps a child thus learn to "aim" his body a bit and develop eye-foot and visual-spatial coordination while also introducing the concept of shapes (e.g., "Let's step on squares only," and so on).

To improve body movement, you can employ a number of useful activities which build upon "simple" walking. Introduce rudimentary counting by having the child step on one square or step on two squares. Introduce directional concepts such as "forward" and "backward," even "sideways" as the child gets the idea. Use shape differences such as step on squares, not circles. Use color; make a game of stopping on green but not red. When other children are present, you can develop the concept of everyone taking turns.

In such ways the fundamental and necessary skills of body movement, including walking, begin to be linked with higher level and more abstract behaviors involving discrimination, balance, and the start of conceptual thinking.

Item 3. Running (circle one)

Date of 1st rating ———— 2nd rating ———— 3rd rating ————

1. Cannot.

2. Needs to hold an adult's hand to run/shuffle along.

3. Unsure and clumsy gait, sometimes fall, but runs independently.

4. Runs fairly well, though still somewhat awkwardly.

5. Runs confidently and gracefully.

Running is a complex skill involving balance and strength. As with walking, the child who is just beginning to learn how to run may need an adult to support her by holding out a hand to steady her. The sheer joy of running tends to be enough to reinforce the pleasure of this activity for most children, though the fun of running with others as well as parental shouts of encouragement add even more fun to learning this skill. Once a child has mastered walking, the activity of running is sure to follow.

As in virtually every activity we discuss, various concepts can be introduced to the child through games involving running. I observed a young mother skillfully introduce various movements or types of running by showing her child how different animals move. Some animals run fast, others run slow; some are graceful, others are *ponderous* (yes, she used that word). She showed him examples of running "lightly" versus running "heavy" (feet go thud, thud, for example). This helps the child discriminate his own movements and, also, to understand how these different movements can be classified. For instance, a person or animal can run powerfully, slowly, quickly, quietly, loudly or ponderously.

In a society in which many children and adults are couch potatoes, encouraging a good conditioning type of activity such as running for fun will benefit your child early in life and later on, as well.

Item 4. Jumping from a height of one foot or more (circle one)

Date of 1st rating _____ 2nd rating _____ 3rd rating _____

1. Unable to do.

2. Can do the jump with considerable adult "lift" or help.

3. Can do the jump with minimal adult help.

4. Jumps alone, but is hesitant and not particularly coordinated at it.

5. Jumps independently with confidence and skill.

Many children, as well as some adults, are fearful of even small heights. However, jumping down from something is often useful to get from one place to another, explore a new place, or just to have fun.

Exposing your child to other children who are jumping down from playground structures, or off boxes or other apparatuses, is always an excellent teaching device. Initially, helping the child by holding his hand may be necessary as he takes his first few jumps. You can eventually wean him from your support by holding his hand with first a lighter and lighter grip, then by having your hand near so that you can offer assistance, if necessary. Once you and the child see that he can jump down on his own, no further adult assistance should be necessary. If the child begs for assistance, it may be that he only wants attention. It is legitimate for little children to desire parental attention, but you don't want to provide reinforcement for the child's dependency, particularly after you know he can do the activity alone. Rather, you would probably do better to keep an eye on the child and be sure to encourage him to try the jump, reinforcing him with delighted praise when he does so. Don't go overboard with this, but some recognition is necessary and nice.

This type of jumping play can be extended and combined with running games or other games. It really depends on the time, patience, and imagination of the parent. The concept of parachutes might be introduced which might lead to talking about "air" and how it can hold a parachute up even though we can't see it. Or, one can use a Jumping Animals game to discriminate between animals that can jump and those that can't. Different types of jumps such as a horse's jump can be compared to a monkey's leap, a baby bird's hop and so on. Of course, activity in the yard or on the playground can then be generalized and applied in some form in the child's room using pictures, books, and stories involving children or animals performing the behaviors such as running or jumping that you and the child did outside.

Item 5. Hopping (circle one)

Date of 1st rating _____ 2nd rating _____ 3rd rating _____

1. Unable to hop.
2. Hops but only with adult help on the "lift" or for balance.
3. Hops alone but hesitantly or clumsily.
4. Hops fairly well alone most of the time, occasionally loses balance.
5. Hops alone confidently and with either foot.

In general, the development of hopping involves the same activities as those used in the development of walking, running and jumping. The same types of activities can be introduced as can the same types of collateral or spin-off concepts. Most children initially hop with two feet at the same time. With a little parental demonstration and assistance, the child can usually quickly learn to hop on one foot a time.

Why do we care about hopping, anyway? Hopping is important as a coordinative activity in its own right in terms of general neuromuscular integration and, also, because it is a forerunner of skipping which involves the smooth contralateral coordination of the body. Contralateral coordination involves initiating activity on one side of the body while inhibiting activity on the other side. Contralateral coordination involves directionality which is related to the development of the inner body feelings of "left" and "right." This physical sense of direction, of left and right, will actually help in the development of reading and writing skills during the early school years.

Item 6. Skipping (circle one)

Date of 1st rating _____ 2nd rating _____ 3rd rating _____

1. Unable to skip.

2. Skips on one side only and needs adult help.

3. Skips on one side though does not need help.

4. Skips on both sides sometimes, though may revert back to one side skipping (hopping).

5. Skips independently with a smooth side to side flow.

The importance of skipping in the development of contralateral coordination and directionality has been noted above. Skipping is a sort of sliding hop. If the child can hop and slide as well as keep her balance on one foot for a moment or so, she should be able to skip. The parent should, of course, make sure that the child can, in fact, hop and slide before attempting to teach her how to skip.

As in many other activities, exposing the child to a peer model who can already skip is a good way to start. Of course, most parents can be models, too; they can skip and demonstrate this activity for the child. Initially, do not be concerned if the child cannot skip at all or skips only on one side. Two-sided skipping should develop with a little practice. As always, do not pressure the child. Allow skipping and other activities to happen easily through enjoyable activities you do together.

Item 7. Use of stairs (circle one)

Date of 1st rating _____ 2nd rating _____ 3rd rating _____

1. Cannot use stairs except to crawl up or bump down on fanny.

2. Can climb up or down one foot by one foot with help.

3. Can use stairs independently but only with same foot first.

4. Alternates feet on successive steps up or down most of the time.

5. Uses stairs independently, holding on to rail or not, using alternate feet all of the time.

The best way for a child to learn how to go up and down stairs is to be around some stairs. If your home does not have stairs, most playgrounds do. Stairs such as those on sliding boards are excellent for novice stair climbers. The movements involved in negotiating up and down stairs aid in development. Also, knowing how to go up and down stairs make the child less likely to get hurt.

Children tend to be able to climb up pretty well, as kittens do, but often run into difficulty coming down. The old fanny-bump technique is usually the first method a child learns. Teach them to bump down feet and fanny first. Some children, however, prefer to sort of crawl down backward. The older child will gradually move from one foot per stair, same foot first to alternating feet while climbing or descending. Facility on the stairs is essentially taught in the same way parents help the child learn to hop, skip and pedal wheel toys. All require contralateral coordination. If the child seems to be having difficulty mastering alternate foot stair use, parents need to take a look at the child's hopping and skipping and other activities requiring foot-leg-eye-brain coordination and practice some of these for awhile.

Item 8. Throwing (circle one)

Date of 1st rating _____ 2nd rating _____ 3rd rating _____

1. Cannot throw a ball or other object.
2. Can throw or push a beach ball; can "toss" a small object by releasing hand (not a true throw).
3. Can throw a ball with underhand or scoop motion in an intended direction.
4. Can throw a ball with underhand or overhand motion, though accuracy is often poor and movements awkward.
5. Can throw a ball either overhand or underhand with good accuracy most of the time.

Ball throwing and catching are excellent ways to develop hand-eye-brain coordination. And, since we live in a culture that likes games, particularly sports using balls, it seems sensible to help the child master ball-playing, at least to some extent.

From a neuromuscular standpoint, the young child is a plastic, malleable being. Her brain development is facilitated by exposure to a wide variety of situations and the ability to master many coordinative skills. When we teach a child to throw, we are helping the child develop coordination between the brain which commands "throw," the eye which perceives where and to what the ball is to be directed, and the child's own hand and arm muscles which will pitch the ball. The child must also come to know when to grip and when to release; he must become familiar with the proprioceptive sense involving touch and feel.

With all this in mind, then, the thoughtful parent will not just give her child a ball and command, "Throw it" when it is his first experience. Rather, the child should be gradually introduced to throwing through use of some large, light ball such as a beachball or even a balloon. Usually, throwing is preceded by the child rolling the ball to you across the rug or the grass. This then progresses to two handed underhand tossing or throwing and on into more refined movements. Rolling and bowling lead to throwing. If the child is having much difficulty throwing a ball to you, tell him to start by walking the ball almost up to your outstretched hands, then releasing it to you. You return the throw in the same manner or by rolling it to him.

As the child is able to toss the ball to you from up close, move farther and farther away as the child's throwing strength, coordination and confidence develops. The procedure of starting with something the child can easily do and then, by gradually moving to more and more elaborated or difficult movements is called *shaping*. Shaping is a useful tool and those who master it tend to be excellent coaches or tutors.

Item 9. Catching (circle one)

Date of 1st rating _____ 2nd rating _____ 3rd rating _____

1. Cannot catch a ball of any size, even from close up.

2. Can catch a beachball though uses a stiff-armed or "clamping" motion.

3. Can catch a beachball if thrower is close and helps child to get set with arms ready.

4. Can usually catch any large- or medium-sized ball in a careful catch and throw game with an adult.

5. Can usually catch any large- or medium-sized ball in any free play situation with an adult or child.

Catching and throwing are like two sides of the same coin. The rationale for catching is similar to that for throwing, the development of eye-hand coordination. However, catching is a little more complex than throwing.

To catch or hit a ball coming toward you your eyes must see that the ball has been thrown and is now coming in your direction. The brain requires accurate information from the eyes to compute the speed and trajectory of the thrown ball. This must happen while another portion of the brain receives this information and, in turn, sends signals out to the relevant muscle groups to position them in an appropriate stance. In short, catching a ball isn't a simple process! This is especially so for the young child whose brain has not yet had the training and programming to enable easy and quick computations of eye to brain muscles.

Although catching and throwing balls is clearly good practice for the brain in terms of information processing, many parents turn their young children off to ball playing because of their lack of consideration of the child's immature brain and the fact that the child may not be developmentally ready to perform the task. The good parent will always go slow.

As with other items, the child's developing skill level is the parent's best guide on how to conduct further training. If children are having a great deal of difficulty learning to catch, use a balloon and initially just bat it back and forth. When the child is able to do this well, you can substitute a large but soft beachball. When he can do this well, use a soft playground-type rubber ball.

When the child is engaged in catching and other similar activities the child's entire brain-body system is literally getting a workout. The smooth functioning of the neuromuscular systems precede and facilitate the development of other cognitive skills.

Item 10. Directionality (circle one)

Date of 1st rating _____ 2nd rating _____ 3rd rating _____

1. Does not know "left" or "right" concepts; cannot follow directions games such as "Simon Says" or left-right directions.

2. Is somewhat able to follow left-right directions but seems generally unsure of self with left-right concepts.

3. Can follow left-right directions fairly well though may often forget and need some coaching.

4. Follows left-right directions well though may need occasional adult help.

5. Seems to have a clear ideas of "left" and "right" and follows left-right directions well.

As discussed, the development of directionality has important implications for the child's acquisition of basic academic skills, especially reading. The Simon Says game is useful because it involves keen discrimination and directional orientation. That is, the child is only supposed to act upon the instructions when the words, "Simon says" precede them. If Simon says, "Raise your left hand" then you do; if the caller only says, "Raise your left hand," then you don't. Other games, such as those involving songs with commands such as, "Put your right foot in," for example, are useful as are games with directions to run to the right, run forward, backward and so on.

Chalkboard drawing, too, will help the child develop directionality as she is encouraged to scribble or draw randomly and shown how to create looping figure eights. Early education specialists note that activities such as copying figure eights on a chalkboard or in sand aids in the development of the child's ability to cross the midline of her body. It also helps perceptual development such as eye tracking and eye-hand coordination, and stimulates the proprioceptive sense. Thus, it combines the sense of touch and sight while assisting in directional training and overall fine and large motor control.

Item 11. Handedness (circle one)

Date of 1st rating _____ 2nd rating _____ 3rd rating _____

1. Not established; child uses either hand indiscriminately; no preferred hand.

2. Poorly established, if at all; child may use one hand for awhile then switch.

3. Fairly well established; usually stays with a preferred hand though not always.

4. Established, although there may be occasional lapses or confusions.

5. Well established; child clearly prefers one hand over the other while drawing, etc.

The remarks pertaining to directionality above also relate to handedness. However, handedness may be established while directionality is not. There is much controversy about what to do if the child has not established a preferred hand on his own by age three years or so. It is not even clear that this is particularly important; however, the child who has established a preferred hand will have more practice in drawing and copying, than the child who splits his practice time by sometimes using his left hand and sometimes his right.

If the child has not developed a preferred hand by age 36 or 40 months, it would be appropriate to start gentle training for right-handedness since we live in a right-handed world. Such training should be as non-intrusive as possible. It involves such things, for example, as handing the child crayons, cups, toys and so on to the right hand. It's all right if the child switches hands, but switch back to the right hand if the child puts the pencil or crayon down. As the child receives more practice trials with the right hand, he'll develop greater proficiency with this hand and have an inclination to increasingly use the more proficient hand. If he's a true "lefty," that's OK. Don't pressure. Teach gently.

CONTROL ON APPARATUS

The child's move from home or backyard play to playground play represents one of the first shifts from the protection of the home environment to the larger world of interaction with other children and, usually, larger pieces of play equipment. Even the casual observer sees the difference between a child who feels capable and comfortable on the sliding boards, swings, tricycles, high platforms and the like of the playground and the timid child who holds back from participating on such equipment. As parents, most of us would prefer to see our child enjoying the equipment and interacting with other children.

It seems wise, as a general rule, to expose the younger child, age two or three years, to smaller equipment in more contained play areas. As the young child becomes accustomed to the smaller sliding boards and other equipment, she'll soon move up to the larger pieces, the higher slides and platforms, with ease and confidence. Introducing the child to water play is useful, too; encourage her but never push beyond her physical or psychological limits.

If a child is inhibited by a piece of equipment, the parent should consider various possibilities. Why should the child feel this way? Is the equipment too large or strange? Is the child's coordination not yet developed enough to use some of the play equipment? If the child seems well-coordinated but fearful, it may be that he may have been pushed too far and too fast by some caretaker in a similar activity and was frightened by the experience. Children tell us when they are not feeling confident or comfortable by hanging back and avoiding the activity.

A child who has been frightened or who may be simply very cautious will often need time to become familiar with play equipment. As stated before, exposure to peers who are using the playground is good strategy because the child can see other children enjoying themselves and thus be encouraged to try the equipment, too. It is pointless to push the cautious child into acting bold. Like some adults, some children need more time to become comfortable with a situation. The suggestions below may help the parent who wants to begin training her child to become competent in various areas but who does not want to pressure or demand complex behaviors before the child is ready.

Item 12. Climbing (circle one)

Date of 1st rating _____ 2nd rating _____ 3rd rating _____

1. Never tries to climb on any of the play equipment.

2. Sometimes tries, but needs considerable help and encouragement.

3. Will try and climb alone to some extent.

4. Climbs on most equipment though may need some help and/or encouragement from time to time.

5. Climbs on all of the equipment, up or down, with competency and confidence.

Climbing about on things, doubtless part of our primate heritage, builds strong arms, shoulders, and backs, develops coordination and promotes confidence in one's body. Most children will climb on their own, needing little encouragement or training. They tend to be able to climb up better than down (as with staircases) so parents may have to help out here. If a child does not climb naturally, the parent must consider whether this is because the child is not developmentally ready for such activity in terms of strength and balance or whether the child is fearful, or some of each.

If the child needs some initial assistance in climbing, the parent should start him at a low level and work up in gradual increments. Interesting climbing games can be devised. Games such as Jack and the Beanstalk links climbing with a well-known story; or the child can pretend to climb imaginary mountains or trees.

Item 13. Balance Beams (circle one)

Date of 1st rating ——————— 2nd rating ——————— 3rd rating ———————

1. Cannot balance on a beam at all.

2. Can balance but needs help all the length of the beam.

3. Can go part of the way without help, though tends to fall off.

4. Usually tries alone and often manages the entire beam without help.

5. Can use the beam freely and walk the length without falling off.

In its simplest form a balance beam is a length of smooth, sanded wood approximately 2″ by 6″ by 72″ or longer. In the home, it is usually laid on a carpeted floor. The dimensions of the beam can be narrowed or broadened depending upon the child's balancing skill. Most people do not have balancing beams (boards) in their homes and many preschools do not have them either. However, a balance beam can greatly assist the development of laterality, directionality and general coordination. Some experts feel that this activity stimulates the sensory integration centers in the brain and facilitates brain-body coordination.

From a neuromuscular view, the balance beam provides the child with a lot of feedback in terms of where her body is, what she needs to quickly do to compensate for leaning one way too far, and how not to overcompensate. This kind of feedback information involves both proprioceptive (inner sensory) and kinesthetic (muscle sensory) elements.

The training is straightforward. Initially you help the child walk the beam. The child may put one foot in front of the other and shuffle along with the same foot first for the length of the beam. Soon, however, the child will be able to place foot over foot on the beam in a more regular walking manner.

Item 14. Slides on the sliding board (circle one)

Date of 1st rating ——————— 2nd rating ——————— 3rd rating ———————

1. Never tries.

2. Tries only with adult help.

3. Occasionally tries alone, though timidly and awkwardly.

4. Usually slides alone, may need encouragement to get started.

5. Uses slide freely in a coordinated manner.

Slides offer good climbing up practice followed by an exciting ride down. The slide down involves balance, including the ability to orient the head and eyes while coordinating overall body movement. Parents can use the slide activity to introduce other concepts such as "up" and "down," waiting in line, safety and so on.

Item 15. Swings (circle one)

Date of 1st rating _____ 2nd rating _____ 3rd rating _____

1. Never uses.

2. Uses only with adult help.

3. Tries to help self into swing and usually can; does not yet "pump" for motion.

4. Can get into swing independently and attempts to pump, though is awkward and ineffectual.

5. Gets into swing alone and pumps strongly, smoothly, and effectively.

Swinging is an excellent stimulus activity for the development of inter-sensory integration. Swinging involves motion, muscles and timing (when to extend legs, when to retract). The parent can also introduce other concepts such as numbers (one, two, three and go) prior to releasing on the first push, or count the pushes out loud once the child is swinging back and forth. You can practice language using directional prepositions such as up and down and adverbs such as fast and slow. Peer models who already know how to "pump" the swing can demonstrate this activity, or the parent can demonstrate it herself. Pumping affords the child more independence since once he can control the activity.

Item 16. Bars and rings (circle one)

Date of 1st rating _____ 2nd rating _____ 3rd rating _____

1. Never uses.

2. Uses only with adult help.

3. Attempts to use but has difficulty grasping and holding on.

4. Can grasp, hang, and support own body weight briefly; cannot go hand over hand.

5. Can grasp, hang, and move hand over hand on the bars or rings independently.

Using the bars or rings on the playground fosters upper body strength and coordination. "Monkey" games are excellent such as swing like a monkey, hang like a monkey. This game can be extended into social participation with peers in a "monkey village" complete with food forays to the ground to get snacks.

Initially, have the child just hold the bar or ring to gradually get used to the idea of supporting his own weight. At a safe height, show him how to let go and drop without hurting himself. After the child has mastered grasping and holding on (this may take a few minutes or a few days or longer, don't hurry it) show him how to swing by giving him a gentle push causing him to sway while he is still holding on. Show him how to slightly loosen his grip to facilitate swaying. Show him how to bend his body at the waist for leverage and back and forth while still hanging on. A child who is introduced to this equipment slowly and safely will soon be jumping, dropping, grasping and swinging—just like a monkey.

Item 17. Wheel toys (circle one)

Date of 1st rating _____ 2nd rating _____ 3rd rating _____

1. Never uses.

2. Uses only with adult help as pusher or holder.

3. Pedals or pushes slowly and has difficulty steering while doing this.

4. Pedals adequately but slowly; sometimes reverses pedaling by mistake and backs up; may sometimes forget to steer.

5. Pedals well, inhibiting one leg while pushing forward with the other and steering accurately at same time.

The importance of contralateral coordination has been discussed above with reference to crawling, walking, skipping, running and walking on the balance beam. Using wheel toys such as tricycles or other pedal toys also develops contralateral coordination. Clearly, contralateral coordination is so important to our proper functioning that most activities develop and train such coordination to some extent.

In general, teaching a child to use wheel or pedal toys is fairly simple. You provide the toy, the child explores it and possibly observes peers using similar toys. You make gentle suggestions as to where the child should place her feet, how to push with one foot while reducing the pressure on the other and so on. Pushing and steering together often require a good deal of practice before the child becomes a competent "driver," so bumping into things is normal at first. Taking turns to use the pedal toy is an obvious adjunctive activity to this one, as is following directions. Many preschools and kindergartens use Stop and Go signs colored red and green, respectively, as part of the instructions. You can put these up at home if you have room for them or you can place directional arrows all around so that all traffic flows in the same direction.

SMALL MUSCLE CONTROL

Physical development of large and small muscle control goes hand in hand with the development of language and symbolic thinking. We understand that the various areas of the child's development is not, in actuality, broken down into the little activity parcels which are presented here. But, in order to enhance physical and mental development, we need to focus on discrete units of behavior. In this section, we'll center our discussion on enhancement of fine motor skills or small muscle coordination.

As is the case with large muscle control, small muscle coordination is activated and enhanced by an environment rich with appropriate learning materials. Most homes and all preschools have plenty of toys and materials—crayons, colored paper, safety scissors, playdo, blocks of all sizes, beads to thread and so on. At home, create a special table or space for the child with these materials where the child can feel free to use them at any time.

Parents will want to provide some structured playtime for the child in which parent and child sit together and both engage in small muscle activities. Parents may like to paint, draw, or build models. Or, you may want to knit, sew or read while your child plays at his table. You may want to write a letter, or a book. After awhile, the child may enjoy being read to at this time, or both of you may enjoy listening to music. You will certainly want to suggest things the child might do, helping out when necessary.

Remember that, initially at least, the child will not know how to use his time well during fine-motor play, a kind of play which, of necessity, tends to be more focused and somewhat quieter and more contained than large muscle activity. Girls often take to the fine motor and focused activities better than boys. But parents should be aware not to force the play table on the boy, or the girl for that matter, if she isn't interested.

All this can be the beginning of a lifelong habit of spending time together, a habit which builds love, empathy, and good communication between you and your child. This bonding will prove to be invaluable later on during the often stressful adolescent years. Perhaps it should also be noted here that this time spent with your child should be free of the television and telephone. Because our society now tends to develop attention deficit disordered people; this, is an opportunity for you to help your child develop small muscle skills as well as the capacity to focus attention on something other than TV or Nintendo for longer and longer periods of time.

Item 18. Stringing beads—defined as placing at least four beads on a shoestring which has a knot tied on the end, by mom or dad (circle one)

Date of 1st rating ———— 2nd rating ———— 3rd rating ————

1. Cannot.

2. Tries, but is clumsy and cannot do but one or two beads, even with adult assistance.

3. Tries and can usually do one or more beads without adult assistance.

4. Can usually do three or four beads without assistance.

5. Can easily string four or more beads without assistance.

Stringing beads seems to be an enjoyable and intrinsically rewarding activity for most children. The fun is extended if the child is provided with sufficient beads to be able to create a necklace or bracelet. Teaching the activity requires little more than providing the material, showing the child how to string a few beads, then allowing the child to do it. The young ones will, of course, need more assistance and larger beads with thicker thread is better. Also, with younger children avoid small beads because of the danger of the child putting them in his mouth and choking.

Bead or block stringing, whether with large or small items, is an excellent activity to develop thumb-finger opposition, eye focusing and hand-eye precision. If you rated your child as Cannot on this activity, encouraging him to stack blocks or play any games involving picking up little things (such as beads) and putting them in a box will be helpful for him.

Item 19. Colors between lines (circle one)

Date of 1st rating _____ 2nd rating _____ 3rd rating _____

1. Cannot.

2. Can do so only with adult help in guiding the crayon.

3. Tries to do so but with poor results, though has the concept of "between lines."

4. Tries to do so and usually manages to stay in lines fairly well.

5. Is fully able to color between lines of a coloring book or her own drawing.

Parents and teachers who place high value on "free expression" may be aghast at our suggestion of training for coloring between lines as soon as a child is reasonably able to do so. Initially, of course, there is no point in insisting that the child color between lines since he simply will not have the fine-motor control to be able to do so. Free form art using scribbles is where most children begin; and this art should be encouraged. We do not want to spoil fun activities such as drawing and coloring by too-quickly insisting that these should be done with precision.

As the child matures and gains more small motor control, he will increasingly be able to put colors between the preset lines of a coloring book. Whether or not young children can color between the large lines of a coloring book is a good means of gauging developing eye-hand dexterity involved with use of paper and pencil (or crayon). Parents should be quite lenient in their interpretation of "between the lines" and, at least initially, offer encouragement for any efforts the child makes that even come close.

For the child rated as Cannot or Can do only with help in guiding the crayon, encourage freehand scribbling with crayon and then move toward more precise or structured coloring by creating an individualized coloring book for the child by drawing only pictures with very large lines, a box or a simple boat, or moon for example. Increase the lines of your drawing until the child can get some colors between them more or less consistently. Then, you can begin to gradually shrink the lines of the figures, but do this slowly, observing carefully at what point you have made the task too difficult for the child's skill level. Once the child appears to have fully mastered coloring between the new lines you have created, shrink these once more and wait for the child's mastery of these and so on. The child learns without frustration or failure because of this gradual shaping method.

Item 20. Drawing a straight line (circle one)

Date of 1st rating _____ 2nd rating _____ 3rd rating _____

1. Cannot.

2. Draws wavy or scribbly lines.

3. Draws crooked lines but seems to have the concept and be attempting to draw a straight line.

4. Draws lines which are more or less straight and about the same length as the line shown to the child to copy.

5. Can draw or copy a straight line on request.

As with coloring between lines, copying a straight line or producing one freehand is another precursor to printing letters and words. Copying a straight line seems simple but actually represents a high degree of eye-hand-brain coordination. Consider the complex brain-body interactions which must take place when the child is requested to draw or copy a line. At a minimum, the child must:

- process the instructions aurally (auditory processing)

- remember the instructions (auditory memory)

- look at the line to be copied (visual attention and perception)

- grasp the crayon (fine motor control)

- send a signal from brain to hand to start drawing (activating the efferent paths of the neuromuscular system)

- receive feedback from hand and eye as to where the crayon is moving (proprioceptive feedback)

- perceive that the line is drawn and cause the hand to stop (inhibition and control of activity).

If the child is having difficulty with line copying or any similar tasks, draw a line in one color and have him copy directly over it with another color. Or, draw two lines about an inch apart and ask the child to place his line between those lines. Another method is to have the child rest his hand on yours as you draw the straight line, then have him try it. For those children who seem to need more help, cut out a sandpaper line and have the child run his fingers over it many times in order to, literally, get the "feel" of the length and form of a straight line by using another sense modality, the sense of touch. Lines (and other shapes, of course) can also be drawn in dirt or sand with the fingers or a stick.

Once the child learns to draw a straight line, you can show him how to make other shapes using similar procedures. The drawing of lines and circles is at about the four-year level on the old form of the Stanford-Binet Intelligence Scale, so don't expect your two or three year old to do this perfectly for awhile.

Item 21. Copying a square (circle one)

Date of 1st rating _____ 2nd rating _____ 3rd rating _____

1. Cannot.

2. Can, but only with an adult guiding her hand.

3. Usually able to copy two or three corners but square may "sag" one way or another.

4. Usually can get three corners right but not exactly a square.

5. Can copy the square, the angles are fine, and it looks like a square.

The general rationale for helping a child learn to copy a square is similar to copying a straight line or other simple shapes. Copying a square is, however, a more complex task than copying a circle or straight line. Nonetheless, all the training techniques noted for assisting a child to learn how to copy a line or other simple shapes are applicable for teaching the copying of a square.

In copying a square, many children manage one or even two angles but often experience difficulty with the other two. A parent can draw half a square and have the child try to complete the rest, or three angles and have the child add the fourth. Have the child observe you copy a square. Talk out loud about what it is you are doing. "We draw a straight line down to here, then go out this way to here, go up to this point and then across to where we started." This is a "thinking out loud" technique which can be used in many different areas with your child.

As the child masters drawing lines, squares, triangles and other shapes show him how to use these to make up things he can draw such as houses, trees, boats and planes. Art stores have simple books of this sort which you can peruse for ideas. Drawing a square is not expected until about the five year level, so don't push your younger child too hard on this.

Item 22. Use of manipulative toys such as Legos (circle one)

Date of 1st rating _____ 2nd rating _____ 3rd rating _____

1. Never tries, uninterested except to pick them up and toss them around.

2. Sometimes sticks pieces together though needs adult direction.

3. Tries independently to put pieces together, has the idea but also has limited success.

4. Can put pieces together adequately in a rather basic way.

5. Can play with the pieces and put them together in creative and innovative ways to make something such as a house, car, for instance.

The ability to use manipulative toys of this kind involves increasing development of fine-motor skills, patience, frustration tolerance and imagination. Such toys are good "mind stretchers." The ability to deal with part-whole relationships is heightened. Creativity, too, can be encouraged. If the child has built many houses and clearly has mastered this bit of construction, ask her to build another house and add something new or ask, "Can you think of anything more we can put on it?" You can also develop pretend games with princes, princesses, kings, and queens or other types of people or creatures. Vocabulary building occurs, too, as you say things such as, "Let's put a *moat* around the *castle*. This will *protect* the people from a *dragon*. A dragon is like a *lizard* but much bigger. They don't really exist but there are pictures of dragons in a book we have which we can look at later."

We hope to assist the child to develop the capacity to create, control, change, and imaginatively explain and discuss his world. Intelligence and imagination arise through the use of manipulables, first in interaction with a skillful parent, then independently for the pure joy of play.

Item 23. Puzzles (circle one)

Date of 1st rating _____ 2nd rating _____ 3rd rating _____

1. Unable to understand the concept of a puzzle; does not attempt.

2. Needs adult help but can do simple two or three piece puzzles.

3. Can work on and usually complete five to eight piece wooden puzzles.

4. Can usually work independently and complete puzzles of eight to twelve pieces or more.

5. Can independently complete puzzles of twenty five pieces or more.

Why would a child or adult enjoy sifting and sorting through various odd shaped pieces of cardboard that, when juxtaposed in a certain way, will represent something? Research with humans and other primates suggests that the mere fact of getting the pieces together is intrinsically rewarding. Just solving problems of almost any kind seems to be enjoyable for most children, as well as adults.

A child who is good with puzzles would be expected to progress to good problem-solving in more complex tasks involving spatial and part-whole relations. At the same time, this activity fosters qualities such as patience, perseverance, and the willingness to try new ways and not get stuck in ruts.

The child needs to be provided with a variety of different kinds of puzzles. He'll start first with the large wooden-piece puzzles of early childhood and progress to the smaller and more complicated puzzles slightly older preschool children play with. If a child seems disinterested in puzzles, consider that the ones he has may be too complex and drop down to a simpler level. At first, you can help the child by linking some pieces yourself and then, to get things started, you might hand the child some pieces showing him where they go.

Many children have no clue as to how to begin a puzzle. Unless you have some other strategy, finding edge pieces first tends to be a good approach. Once the edge or frame of the puzzle is completed, show the child how to look for similar pieces such as parts of a house or face, and how to use color cues. The ability to deal with subtle cues will greatly assist the child later when she is in school and needs to follow directions, derive information from embedded text and many other academic activities.

Item 24. Use of pencils and crayons (circle one)

Date of 1st rating ——————— 2nd rating ——————— 3rd rating ———————

1. Cannot grasp even to scribble or has no interest or understanding of pencil/crayon.

2. Can scribble, grasping crayon full-handed and awkwardly.

3. Can make rudimentary shapes or scrawl some designs given some assistance.

4. Can copy or create various shapes fairly well, needs some adult assistance.

5. Holds pencil/crayon between thumb and forefingers and draws/colors well.

Initially, most children grasp the pencil/crayon with the whole hand, fingers wrapped entirely around the shaft. In the normal course of events and through much practice and opportunity to use pencils/crayons, this activity is refined until the child is able to hold the crayon with thumb and forefingers correctly, arm rested on table, body angled slightly toward the work on the table or floor and eyes following movements of arm and hand. As with all complex behaviors, use of pencil/crayons involves many simpler behaviors. As a rule, when a child is having difficulty with any complex activity, analyze the simpler sets of behaviors that underlie the activity. If you can spot what is not yet learned, teach the simpler behavior, for instance, holding the pencil more adequately, then resume teaching the complex behavior.

Item 25. Page turning (circle one)

Date of 1st rating ——————— 2nd rating ——————— 3rd rating ———————

1. Cannot.

2. Turns pages one or several pages at a time with assistance.

3. Usually turns one page at a time without assistance and usually without tearing the page.

4. Can turn pages one at a time, though occasionally may turn several at once.

5. Fully able to turn one page at a time in a left to right direction, let go and not tear, and do this without adult help.

Page turning is clearly a useful activity to help your child learn, otherwise many of your books and hers may have their pages ripped out. Page turning behavior involves thumb and first finger in opposition as well as a delicate grasp and release. The child must perceive when to release using kinesthetic or sense of touch discrimination in learning the "feel" of the activity.

Problems with page turning came to my attention many years ago while I was engaged in a project involving pre-kindergarten and kindergarten age children from very deprived backgrounds. Many of these children, we found, had never held a book in their hands before. They did not know how to turn a page. They could not seem to sense when to grasp and when to release; nor did they know in what direction to turn a page. These behaviors and many others had to be taught to these children before we could even begin to address their basic academic learning.

Item 26. Use of scissors (circle one)

Date of 1st rating _____ 2nd rating _____ 3rd rating _____

1. Unable to use.

2. Needs help inserting fingers into the open handle and scissoring.

3. Tries independently but usually needs help to actually cut paper.

4. Fairly competent, though may need help to cut out a certain shape.

5. Uses scissors very adequately, can cut along a straight line and/ or cut out shapes as requested or as she desires.

The appropriate use of scissors clearly involves excellent fine-motor control and perceptual integration. Among other things, using scissors involves the ability to squeeze thumb and forefinger together while also grasping firmly to prevent the scissors from slipping from one's grasp. The other hand, meanwhile, must hold a piece of paper or other material in such a manner that the scissors can easily cut through it.

As with other activities, the ability to learn how to use scissors generally depends upon how accessible this tool is to her (use only the blunt safety scissors), whom the child sees using such equipment and how motivated she may be to participate in the activity. To train to use scissors, show the child how scissors work and what they do; help her slip her fingers into the handle, then move the child's fingers slowly up and down to form the cutting motion using your own

fingers on the scissors with the child's. In this way, she can get the feel
of the activity.

   If, after introductory training, the child still cannot use scissors well
or perhaps not at all, then consider the possibility that one or more
of the various fine motor or perceptual antecedents leading up to the
complex behavior of using scissors has not yet been well-developed.
Can the child string beads (thumb and forefinger opposition required)? Can she turn pages? Can she perceive lines and shapes in
order to cut along the design? If not, drop back and teach the simpler
behaviors once more, then come back later to training for the use of
scissors.

Item 27. Folding paper (circle one)

Date of 1st rating _____ 2nd rating _____ 3rd rating _____

   1. Cannot.

   2. Can fold one piece over once awkwardly and needs assistance.

   3. Folds more or less randomly, not precisely, but seems to know
      what "fold" means and is trying to do so.

   4. Can fold vertically and/or horizontally.

   5. Can fold a piece of paper vertically, horizontally or diagonally
      and can fold over fold.

   With the exception of newspaper delivery boys or girls or paper
airplane aficionados, folding paper would not appear at first glance to
be a particularly useful or requisite skill. However, folding paper does
require neuromuscular skills, perceptual activity, and, ultimately,
some planning or forethought. And, beyond the mastery of one more
set of coordinative activities, folding paper involves some thinking
activity. For instance, where does the clown's face go when you fold
the paper? Does it disappear? Is it under the fold? Or, we can fold the
paper and make an airplane or a boat or hat. And, by so doing we've
created a toy which we did not have to purchase at the toy store.

Item 28. Dressing (circle one)

Date of 1st rating _____ 2nd rating _____ 3rd rating _____

   1. Cannot.

   2. Needs much adult help but can get some clothes partially on or off.

3. Needs much adult help but can get most clothes on or off.

4. Needs some adult help but for the most part can dress self.

5. Dresses self independently (with the possible exception of tying shoes).

Having the ability to dress herself is a useful and desirable skill for the child to learn. She feels more grownup and independent. You feel relief at having one less task to do. In learning to dress, the child is, of course, initially clumsy and lacks coordination or even the prior thought about what clothes she will put on. Because there is so much involved, the parent introduces the idea of dressing gradually. Start with showing the child the relatively easy tasks such as putting on socks, then perhaps velcro tennis shoes. Show her how to put feet in pants or a dress over the head, and move on up to more difficult items such as shirts or coats in which one has to figure out how to get arms through and/or get over the head.

In all phases of teaching the child how to dress herself we move from the simple to the more complex. Initially, the child will need much assistance. Be sure to provide this without fussing or showing frustration. Help the child every step of the way. Use a "thinking out loud" technique and match what you are doing with the child to your words. "Your arm goes here, now the other arm over here in this sleeve, then we pull the shirt right over your head and it's on. Hooray!"

Children acquire the skill of dressing themselves at different rates, but they all eventually master it. Continue walking the child through the procedures, this helps him literally get the feel (kinesthetic feedback) for how to move when dressing and what sequence to use. Speak in a gentle tone throughout the process. "We are putting your right leg into your pants, now your left leg. When you see both feet sticking out at the bottom, you then stand up and pull your pants on."

Some children may balk at dressing themselves and continue to want you to do this for them. When this happens, analyze the situation carefully. Is it that the child has not yet learned the components of dressing herself and is still struggling with this task? Or, does dressing herself possibly mean, to her mind, that soon she will be leaving mom and going off to preschool? Or, is wanting to be dressed by mom or dad a regression to a more babyish state and, possibly, a desire for more parental attention.

If the child has not yet developed the coordination for dressing herself, continue working with her on the fundamental components until she has mastered them. If the child is balking because of school, talk with her teacher and find out if something unpleasant is happening there. If the child is being somewhat manipulative and attempting to get more of your attention, carefully consider whether or not she is getting sufficient individual time with you. If you are not sure, provide the child with more of your time and attention in positive activities, thus precluding the need for her to attempt to gain your attention in a negative manner such as refusal to dress or other negative behaviors.

Item 29. Buttoning (circle one)

Date of 1st rating _____ 2nd rating _____ 3rd rating _____

1. Cannot.

2. Only with considerable help.

3. Can get button partially through the hole.

4. Manages alone most of the time, though only partially succeeds and often needs help.

5. Can get his clothes buttoned with no help.

In order to button, one must be able to "pinch" a button (thumb-forefinger opposition), guide it to the buttonhole, twist it sideways, then slip it through the buttonhole. Behaviorally, this is very complicated. So, before suggesting that the child dress himself and button his clothes, you should be certain that she can perform all the "little" behaviors that go to make up the whole of this complex behavior called buttoning. If you feel that she cannot do these little behaviors, help her learn them; if you are fairly sure she can do them, then just go ahead and show her how to button while talking out loud about holding it, twisting it, slipping it through.

There are buttoning materials available at children's stores. These usually involve pieces of cloth, some with buttons and some with buttonholes. The buttons are large and usually brightly colored, the buttonholes may be cut slightly larger than would be usual in order to make the child's initial practice easier.

Gentle verbal encouragement is the appropriate method to use with almost all tasks which children are learning. When teaching, you can add a comment such as, "You are doing well. Soon, you will be able to button all your clothes yourself." Avoid an exasperated tone as in, "When will you ever learn how to do this?" As a general rule, when a child is not learning a given task quickly it is either because the parent or teacher has not figured out an effective manner of teaching it, or the child is not yet developmentally able to do the task.

BLADDER AND BOWEL CONTROL

Item 30. Bladder control (circle one)

Date of 1st rating _____ 2nd rating _____ 3rd rating _____

1. No control.

2. Frequent lapses, still needs diapers.

3. Occasional lapses, may need diapers or training pants depending on the situation.

4. Adequate control, though often needs reminders to relieve self.

5. Full control, urinates independently when the need arises, rarely needs reminders.

In the ordinary course of life, children move from no control to reliable control of their bladder during the first five years or so. However, children age six and older may have occasional lapses, especially during sleep, for years.

With younger children, training for control primarily involves observing the child's usual time of urinating and putting him on a routine so he can gradually urinate on demand. That is, he is "toileted" at more or less regular intervals. If the child becomes accustomed to relieving himself every hour or so, he will begin to put himself on his own schedule. The young child will need to be placed on a baby toilet or regular toilet with a baby attachment at regular intervals until he can urinate voluntarily when on the toilet and withhold urination when not on the toilet.

Parents should offer gentle and restrained encouragement for the child's use of the toilet. Toilet training tends to be of great concern for many parents. They want to accomplish this fairly soon since many preschools will not admit untrained children. An excellent book about this subject is *Toilet Training In Less Than A Day* by the psychologists Nathan Azrin and R.M. Foxx.[1] A useful companion book by Nathan Azrin and Victoria Besalel is *A Parent's Guide to Bedwetting Control.*[2]

Item 31. Bowel control (circle one)

Date of 1st rating _____ 2nd rating _____ 3rd rating _____

1. No control.

2. Frequent lapses, diapers still necessary.

3. Occasional lapses, can use training pants fairly safely.

4. Adequate control most of the time, can and will get on toilet for bowel movement.

5. Full control, goes to the toilet regularly when needs to move bowels.

The remarks regarding training for bladder control (above) are, for the most part, also relevant for training bowel control. A major difference between bladder and bowel elimination, of course, is that the child usually needs to be cleaned more carefully after a bowel movement. Most young children do not clean themselves well, at least initially.

Parents as well as preschool teachers tend to be more concerned about a child's soiling than wetting, especially if the child is four or older. If the child has not established adequate bowel control by this age, this should be discussed with your pediatrician. If the child has been trained and has regressed to soiling again (and/or wetting) this, too, should be discussed with your doctor. It could represent some psychological disturbance that may happen after the birth of a sibling, or as a reaction to separation from mother or home upon being enrolled in preschool, or because of factors such divorce of parents.

Do not be too quick, however, to interpret such behavior or to react to it. Wetting and soiling regressions are not uncommon among young children. Control has only been minimally developed at this age, and various stressors in the child's life may easily override the newly learned ability to control his bladder or bowels. If there is regressive loss of control, go back to your initial training regimen with the child. If the loss of control continues, consult with your pediatrician or a psychologist who specializes with young children.

In the next chapter, we start with two kinds of memory functions and then proceed to problem-solving as well as many items having to do with the critically important language functions. It is important to note that the items in this book are *not* necessarily ordered in terms of importance with, say, Item 1 or 15 or 36 being somehow more important than item 37 or 45, for instance.

I believe that every item in this book represents some aspect which is important with respect to a balanced development of the child. Once more, I remind parents to remember that they are cautioned against "testing" the child on any item and, further, parents should not be disturbed if your child's development is uneven and she is stronger in some areas than in others. Uneven development is characteristic of early childhood and to be expected. It will not be until the "five year to seven year shift" (Chapter 12) that we will begin to expect and witness smoother performance across almost all areas of development for most children.

NOTES

1. Azrin, N.H. and Foxx, R.M. *Toilet Training In Less Than A Day*. New York: Simon and Schuster. 1974.
2. Azrin, N.H. and Besalel, V.A., *A Parent's Guide to Bedwetting Control*. New York: Pocket. 1979.

9

The Foundations of Higher Order Thinking

Memory, Language, Basic Cognitive Skills, Self-Awareness and Problem Solving

While exploring all the ways to develop the intelligence of our children, memory is a critically important subject to consider. The different aspects of memory, when linked with the nuances and power of language, are the prime underpinning of human intelligence. As with other human skills, memory and language both require certain environmental conditions before they can develop; to *fully* develop, they need enrichment stimulation from a kind and thoughtful parent.

Basic cognitive skills involving the use of colors, shapes, letters, awareness of cause-effect relationships and rudimentary problem solving are usually more widely promoted in our society than the memory and language skills mentioned above. Everywhere we turn—in a children's store or educational supply outlet we see activities involving letters, shapes and numbers. The development of these skills is clearly important but, it is again noted, they *follow* the development of basic memory and language skills.

MEMORY

Item 32. Recognition Memory (circle one)

Date of 1st rating _____ 2nd rating _____ 3rd rating _____

1. None apparent, child does not appear to recognize familiar faces, objects or sounds.

2. Minimal recognition of familiar faces, objects or sounds (for example, seems to recognize faces of parents but is much more uncertain about others).

3. Fair recognition of familiar faces or objects but may be lapses unless there is frequent contact.

4. Good recognition of faces, objects (a toy), or sounds (a particular melody), though there may be some lapses.

5. Excellent recognition of familiar faces, objects, names, sounds with no lapses.

Recognition is one of the most basic forms of memory. Infants recognize familiar faces, sounds, smells and objects very early in life. As the infant's brain and nervous system develop in conjunction with muscle systems that allow for bodily movement including grasping, putting objects in mouth, crawling then standing and walking and so on, "recognition memory" expands. After this memory is developed the infant will have the ability to recognize shapes, colors, numbers, letters, sound sequences, as well as story themes and pictures.

The infants recognition memory will more or less develop on its own in most circumstances. However, there are ways to enhance this skill. You can let him see a lot of faces of friends and relatives. The peek-a-boo game gives him an added dimension of pleasure and makes him smile when he recognizes people. Show him photographs of family members and friends to help establish and expand his recognition memory. Regularly playing particular songs, rereading selected stories and playing of carefully chosen children's videos is helpful, too. When appropriate, parents can expand the infants basic recognition memory by talking about or naming people, places and objects.

If your child seems to exhibit very poor recognition memory, discuss this with your pediatrician.

Item 33. Language-Based Recall Memory (circle one)

Date of 1st rating _____ 2nd rating _____ 3rd rating _____

1. None apparent. Cannot yet recall location of her eyes, nose, teeth and does not yet, for example, respond to questions such as "Show me your nose" or "Where are your teeth."

2. Basic language is present and child can recall or say own name, find her nose, teeth, and so on.

3. Can recall and say names of family members, relatives, and playground friends.

4. Good recall and can say names of family, relatives, preschool or neighborhood friends.

5. Good recall and can verbally recite recent events, names, home address or phone number, names of teachers or neighbors and so on.

Recall memory is more difficult than simple recognition memory. Recall memory is involved when the child is asked a question or requested to do something based on previous learning. For example, to the baby, "Where is your nose?," or "Bring me the Lion King book," to the toddler. With the preschooler, "What is your teacher's name?" There are two aspects of recall memory—short-term and long-term.

Short-term recall memory involves the vitally important aspects auditory and visual memory. There is also, of course, olfactory, kinesthetic and proprioceptive memory but here we are focusing on the forms of memory most important for academic success. Adequate auditory memory enables the child to do such things as remember sounds in sequences such as the ABCs, simple directions or even several directions given in sequence—get your book, get your coat, wait by the door. Adequate visual memory enables the child to recall a sequence of visual stimuli, the details of a picture, or the story line of a movie he has recently seen. Short-term recall is useful since it enables us to act effectively in the here and now. We can recall a phone number we used just a few minutes ago, and we can remember the directions to the freeway in a strange town. This information remains in short-term or, as it has more recently been termed, working memory until it is no longer useful. There is no reason to clutter up long-term memory (we'll get to this soon) with bits of information for which only short-term memory is required. Short-term memory helps us move efficiently through our days, and is important for another reason, as well. If information is not taken into short-term memory (auditory or visual or both), it cannot be processed to long-term memory storage.

Enhancing short-term memory involves working with the child to exercise immediate recall with activities such as "Listen to what I say and say it after me." "Watch what I do and then copy me," for example. You can stretch sequences longer, "Now watch three things I'm going to do and then you do them." Hiding games are good sources of memory training and fun. The child looks at two, then three or four things. Have him look away, then remove one item. Ask him to tell you which one is missing.

The development of longer-term memory (recall memory) is achieved when you ask questions about what you did yesterday, last week; what you did on last summer's vacation. As mentioned in the section on recognition memory, a family album of photos is a good technique here, too, as are videos recorded on vacations. Be sure to discuss these cherished memories at other times when she is not viewing the photos or videos.

Memory and intelligence go hand in hand. The memory functions, short-term and long-term, auditory and visual, are virtually the foundations of intelligence. Good memory functions are a necessary, though not entirely sufficient, condition for high level intellectual performance (language functions must also be well-developed).

Some children's short-term memory can be adequate and long-term memory rather poor, or vice versa. As discussed earlier, if information is not efficiently processed through short-term memory it cannot be "transferred" to long-term memory for storage. Some children process information so slowly that little goes to short-term memory, thus creating difficulties in long-term memory. School age children who manifest difficulty in short- or long-term memory, either in the visual or auditory modalities, may experience much frustration when they start school and encounter formal teaching procedures. If your kindergarten or first grade age child seems to be having such difficulties, do not use this or any other book to assess the problem. Rather, discuss the matter with your pediatrician, the school psychologist, or a child psychologist who specializes in diagnostic work with learning problems.

LANGUAGE

Like memory, language is vitally important to intellectual functioning. Effectively using language depends upon the child's ability to hear, process, and then respond to sounds made by people or things. There are two major divisions of language, receptive and expressive, with sub-divisions in each. It is extremely important that the child understand incoming sounds, for without this ability no further language development can occur. Therefore, our discussion will initially focus on receptive language.

A REMINDER

Please recall the manner in which the BARI is used. It is expected that infants and young children will be rated low. This is not of concern since they are not developmentally ready for many things. For example, in the item below, it is normal for infants, for example, to have no actual understanding of words (though they recognize familiar sounds). This will quickly change, however, as the child develops some basic understanding of sounds and begins to discriminate them increasingly effectively. This kind of development will be the case for all BARI items, not just language-based items.

Item 34. Receptive Language I—understanding speech of others (circle one)

Date of 1st rating _____ 2nd rating _____ 3rd rating _____

1. No apparent understanding of words though responds to familiar sounds.

2. Appears to have some rudimentary understanding of a few words, for example, and will point to body parts such as nose or eyes upon request.

3. Seems to understand and tries to act upon basic commands such as, "Hand me the ball," though may need repeated requests.

4. Understands simple sentences and commands as well as more complex directions such as, "Go up to your room and get the pictures that you drew in your new coloring book."

5. Clearly understands both simple and complex sentences or phrases whether these are in the form of directions, instructions or explanations.

A developing baby *in utero* can respond to sounds as clearly as a newborn. Thus, a young child should be highly responsive to sounds.

In this early stage of life baby and young child begin to make sense out of the various sounds; they process them and, eventually, remember them (see previous section on memory). Receptive language involves processing efficiency as well as the ability to focus on sounds. Generally, children get a lot of practice in their early lives as they listen to questions and comments from parents and other adults. Playing games with verbal clues—now you're getting warmer, now colder; catch the ball, come here—help develop receptive language skills.

More advanced receptive language skills will involve listening to stories, following complex directions, enjoying music and so on. These skills will become very important when the child learns phonics as he develops reading skills in school.

Item 35. Receptive Language II—ability to follow verbal directions (circle one)

Date of 1st rating _____ 2nd rating _____ 3rd rating _____

1. Shows no ability at all in following verbal directions.

2. Can do but only with strong adult involvement such as gestures, repetitions.

3. Tries to do so but often does not understand or does so imperfectly.

4. Usually understands and follows verbal directions successfully.

5. Fully capable; understands and follows verbal directions.

This category obviously has much overlap with Item 34 above. Unless a child is able to focus on and act upon verbal directives he is not fully open and ready for a more extensive enrichment education. In our culture so much of our interaction with children involves language directives of one sort or another, for example, the parental, "Watch how I do it"; "Listen, now . . ."; "Let's sit down here." "When everyone is quiet, I'll read you a story."

Some children are not yet developmentally able to process, remember, and respond to verbal instructions, others simply will not follow directions very well. For the children who are developmentally immature and have not yet developed "following verbal directions" skills, the same types of games and activities suggested for Item 34 should be helpful. If the child does not want to please an adult and thus follow directions, consider the following points. The child may have been turned off to verbal directions, perhaps because too many such directives were uttered too soon in the child's life. Or, there were no consequences at all when the child followed directions, requests or commands. In other words, the adult was ineffectual in communicating with the child and the child learned little or nothing about following adult verbal directions. If you feel that this may be the case with your child, go to a resource book such as Gerald Patterson's *Living With Children*[1] and acquaint yourself with some simple, but effective techniques that will help you gently and quickly change this situation.

Essentially, you will want to practice saying what you mean and meaning what you say. Providing some mildly negative consequence when the child does not follow directions, and granting some pleasant consequence (your approval or a hug) when your child obeys. Don't reinforce the negative. Don't get caught up in fussing with the child about not following directions, the child may be getting a lot of negative attention out of this. Be sure you are providing enough positive attention when the child is being an OK kid.

Item 36. Receptive Language III—listening and response to stories (circle one)

Date of 1st rating ———— 2nd rating ———— 3rd rating ————

1. No apparent response.

2. Listens for very short periods; may answer a direct question about the story.

3. Listens for longer periods, may need adult guidance to focus on the story.

4. Likes stories and will usually listen and respond to story discussion.

5. Likes stories and will usually listen with good interest and ask questions or make comments spontaneously.

From our discussion about ability to respond to verbal directives, we move into the area that provides so much satisfaction for humans—the ability to listen with discrimination and for pleasure. From this ability stems the child's capacity for relating sequences of words, phrases, sounds, ideas in meaningful way. Auditory processing and auditory memory are used, of course, as is imagery and imagination. To be able to listen to a story is a wonderful ability, opening the child to being touched by another's use of language which in turn stimulates her imagination. Jim Trelease, in his *Read Aloud Handbook*, offers parents many stories appropriate for different age groups and suggests many do's and don'ts when reading to your child.[2] Trelease suggests that you initially read your child stories that you enjoy yourself, but don't continue reading once it is obvious that the book is a poor choice. Also, you should not read above the child's emotional level; be careful, too, about rushing through a story. It's better not to start reading if you are not going to have enough time to do the story justice.

"Listening" is a highly complex skill built upon other, more fundamental skills such as ability to focus, emotional readiness to sit still and to understand the concept of "story being read" and the already-noted auditory processing and memory skills. To make matters more complicated, in order for a child to be a "good listener" much depends upon who is reading the story, the story itself, whom the child is sitting next to, how tired or hungry the child is and so on. Since being able to be quiet, comfortable and attentive is a learned skill, parents will want to start reading to their child when she is very young and continue reading until the child becomes an accomplished reader herself. Indeed, many adults enjoy hearing a good story either read or told to them.

Read to the child without the competing sounds of the radio or TV. If parents are just beginning this program, realize that the modern TV-oriented child may not want to sit still and listen but, rather, prefers computer games or TV. Parents have to help the child acquire a love of listening by not only reading the stories to him while insisting that TV be shut off, but also by introducing him to reading groups at the library or local school or bookstore.

Item 37. Language-articulation (circle one)

Date of 1st rating _____ 2nd rating _____ 3rd rating _____

1. Not understandable at all.

2. Mumbles, whines, or baby talks to the extent that it's difficult understanding what the child is saying.

3. Uses understandable single words but rarely or never uses full and understandable sentences.

4. Usually understandable though may use occasional words or phrases which are not easily understood.

5. Speaks clearly; anyone listening can understand all words and phrases.

The formation of the series of complex sounds that we call intelligible speech first involves adequate development of certain areas of the brain. It also requires the ability to hear and to discriminate sounds, adequate language models on which we pattern our own speech, and differential reinforcement for certain sounds which, of course, eventuates in the varying languages we find among different peoples of the world.

As a consequence of the complexities involved in the child's development of the production of clear and understandable sounds parents should take a tolerant and low-keyed view toward "speech teaching." Clear speech is not so important as is the child's attempting to speak. We first need to encourage the child to make sounds, then later we slowly and patiently assist the child to develop clearer, more precise speech. In general, it is probably better that parents and other adults adhere to their own speech standards when speaking with a child, but refrain from correcting his early and imprecise speech. The child will naturally mimic your speech over time, though some sounds may be difficult for him for a while. With infants, of course, "motherese" is the preferred communication method on the part of the parent though at that stage, the child is generally not at a point of articulating words himself.

Item 38. Expressive Language (circle one)

Date of 1st rating _____ 2nd rating _____ 3rd rating _____

1. Does not express self in words, uses cries, grunts or gestures.

2. Uses a few words or two-word sentences (Have cookie?).

3. Can make simple statements and ask simple questions.

4. Offers more complex statements and questions (When is daddy coming home?).

5. Freely engages in questioning and answering, carries on a basic conversation.

Although the ability to recognize and remember visual and auditory stimuli is impressive, our ability to express ourselves verbally ranks as one of the more important developmental achievements of the human being. Language, in the form of spoken words is a uniquely human attribute. A major part of intellectual development is the capacity to translate thoughts, memories, and feelings into words, then into connected words in sentences, then into longer groups of words and ideas, a process called connected discourse. Writing, a second order language function, is built on the foundation of expressive language.

Most child development specialists now agree that language is a dormant attribute in all physically normal human children, needing only appropriate stimulation for development. Since almost all children the world over receive at least some language stimulation, most of us learn to talk and to express ourselves reasonably well with language. Listening to conversation and stories helps develop receptive language and lays the groundwork for expressive language.

As we've said before, some TV programs such as Sesame Street, for instance, can help children develop language skills. But, we want to emphasize that there is no better coach, tutor and developmental/intellectual skill-builder than an intelligent, loving and interested parent.

BASIC COGNITIVE SKILL DEVELOPMENT

Colors, shapes, numbers and letters

Item 39. Use of Colors (circle one)

Date of 1st rating _____ 2nd rating _____ 3rd rating _____

1. Dabbles or "messes" with paints but cannot name or recall colors.

2. When shown a color, can usually name or point to objects of similar color in the room.

3. Can name and select two or three colors when requested to do so or can point to something of that color.

4. Can name most or all of the more common or frequent colors, for instance, the primary colors, on request.

5. Can name all familiar or primary colors and can recall colors of various toys or other aspects of the environment such as the color of the sky or the color of grass.

Identifying colors relates to other abilities having to do with using crayons as well as recognition, and recall. However, it is an important subject and deserves to be discussed here. Color knowledge plays an important part in preschool and, of course, the child is expected to be fully color aware by the time he enters kindergarten. Apart from the magic of seeing how primary colors blend into secondary colors, how sunlight "breaks up" into all the colors of the rainbow when passed through a prism, and how changing the illumination in a room alters perceived coloration, color naming and general color knowledge is important as a communicative function in the early years (the blue sky; the red car; the brown dog). Reasonably accurate color perception sharpens and enriches the child's ability to understand what he sees, relate it to what he hears, and to enjoy his world more expansively. Color knowledge and color awareness expand the child's perceptual boundaries.

Item 40. Shapes (circle one)

Date of 1st rating ————— 2nd rating ————— 3rd rating —————

1. No seeming awareness of shapes, jumbles blocks or pieces of puzzles together; does not know square from round, for example.

2. Can point to and/or match simple shapes.

3. Recognizes basic shapes; can point to a square, circle, triangle.

4. Can sort out the basic shapes from an assortment.

5. Can do all of the above plus create basic shapes by drawing them or creating them out of clay or similar material.

This item is related to Item 22 (Copies various shapes and symbols) but there are important differences between the two. Item 22 emphasizes the fine-motor coordination involved in copying shapes and symbols. This item emphasizes the child's understanding of the concept of "different shapes." That is, the child can distinguish and define the shape of a square as opposed to that of a triangle and so on. We assume that the child has the concept of, say, "squareness" if the child can sort out and discriminate squares from other shapes, name squares when she sees them and when asked to do so, draw a square, and explain how a square is different from a circle or triangle.

The concept of shape is taught, as are all other concepts such as the concept of self, of rules and so on. We instruct from the concrete all the way to the abstract. We start with the basic notion of "shape" and the fact that all things have shape. Using a red ball, for example, we immediately integrate the interrelated concepts of "redness," "ballness," and "roundness." There are few pure concepts at this concrete level. You explain the concept of round using words and gestures. You compare the round ball with the square block, one rolls the other does not; one has sharp angles or edges, the other has no angles or edges and so on. You can walk around with your child, asking her to look around the room for other round things such as other round balls, round stones, round pumpkins or oranges, and almost-round apples or peaches. You again emphasize the qualities that make things round, then have her practice the fine-motor activity of drawing round things, cutting out round circles or balls.

Item 41. Numbers—counting (circle one)

Date of 1st rating _____ 2nd rating _____ 3rd rating _____

1. No apparent awareness of the concept of "number."

2. Can "count" objects up to one or two and seems dimly aware of the concept of number at this level.

3. Can count three to ten or more items but must rely on tangible aids such as blocks to do so.

4. Can count to ten or so without tangible aids; can go higher with tangible aids.

5. Can count to twenty or more without tangible aids; understands the concept of number.

This item relates to the child's ability to say, "One, two, three…" in sequence, to count in merely a rote fashion and truly understand numbers and that they represent an amount of something.

Over the years, many ways have been devised to teach counting. That is no great feat since horses, pigeons and goldfish have been taught elementary counting "skills." It is, however, another matter to teach the child the concept of number. Math is a powerful thinking tool. When the child grasps the concept that a bunch of something has a number, that things added to or taken away from the bunch change the number we assign to the bunch, and so on, she is beginning to develop the ability to think and to manipulate the most abstract of abstracts—numbers.

The parent would be wise to always gently and non-intrusively pair the abstract term with concrete examples. "There are two elephants here. Oh, look, over there is the baby elephant. That makes three elephants here." This will help the child move from the concrete sights and sounds which surround her to the abstract notions of more and less and number assignment and manipulation, the very stuff of higher order math abstractions. Just as a language experience approach involves reading to the child and surrounds her with words to hear, say, look at and copy, so should a math approach attempt to surround the child with numbers and things to count and measure. You can also introduce her to the use of number words and number ideas. For example, ask questions such as, "How many would you say a lot of children would be? and so on.

Item 42. Number Recognition (circle one)

Date of 1st rating _____ 2nd rating _____ 3rd rating _____

1. No apparent awareness or recognition of number printed, drawn or spoken.

2. Recognition of a number as a number, even though may be inaccurate (May say "one" when presented with two things).

3. Can recognize one or two of the basic numbers such as 1, 2, or 3 when spoken or when seen in a picture book.

4. Can recognize single numbers 1 though 9.

5. Can recognize all the single numbers as well as the double numbers up to 20.

As in Item 41, the heart of the matter is the development of number concept or number awareness. The focus of this item, however, is the child's recognition of numbers when he sees them printed on a chalkboard, on paper or in one of his storybooks. Just as we teach the ABCs, we want to teach number counting. The single digits require the memorization of nine numbers, obviously (Teach zero and the concept of zero later). After the child has mastered the recognition and recall of the nine single-digit numbers, advance to the double-digit numbers up to 20. This involves 11 more number combinations for the child to learn. All of this is going on with the continued, gentle immersion of the child in math (and language) real-world experience. The ability to recognize and eventually recall numbers and letters enhances the child's conceptual development and lays the groundwork for academic skills.

Item 43. Letters—recognition and recall (circle one)

Date of 1st rating _____ 2nd rating _____ 3rd rating _____

1. None apparent.

2. Can recognize and/or recall or say first three letters (ABC) though probably not much real grasp of what they mean.

3. Can say most of the letters of the alphabet; can recognize letters in own name.

4. Can say all or most of the alphabet with assistance of prompts such as rhyming songs, with little help from parent; can consistently recognize letters of own name as well as some words.

5. Can say the alphabet upon request; can recognize all of the letters of the alphabet.

Recognition and recall could each have their own item, of course, but here we combine them because that is more or less how they are taught, in combination. Recognition of letters involves the child's ability to name the letter when it is presented on a paper, in a book and so on. Recall of letters involves the child's ability to say the ABCs without having the letters in front of him. In general, children learn to recognize and recall the first few letters of the ABCs rather easily, probably because they are presented with them so often in books and songs. It's important to note the obvious but significant fact that recognition is not recall but precedes recall.

Immerse your child in letters and numbers and language in a gentle way. Compare it to giving him a bubble bath. We don't "teach" the child to enjoy the bath, but most children do. We don't need to "teach" letters and numbers and concepts either. Just put them all around the child and let him, as with a bath, soak in them often.

Item 44. Letters—printing (circle one)

Date of 1st rating _____ 2nd rating _____ 3rd rating _____

1. Cannot.

2. Can legibly copy some letters of his own name or other letters.

3. Can legibly copy letters of his own name as well as most other letters, if not all.

4. Can print letters of own name without copying.

5. Can print any letter without copying, though may not yet be able to spontaneously print the entire alphabet.

Writing serves as a major stepping stone to reading. A child prints before he learns cursive so when we speak of writing we are talking about printing. Since children are now often introduced to computers at an early age, the child should be led toward typing and the use of a word processing program as soon as possible.

For most children, learning the ABCs and their own name serves as an introduction to reading and writing. Clearly, since adequate co-ordination is involved, we do not want the child to be trying to write before she has mastered the basic eye-hand coordinative skills involved (see Chapter 7). However, assuming adequate coordina-tive skills which enable the child to grasp the pencil, sit in an erect manner, position the paper, and so on we can begin to teach writing.

The first form of writing is scribbling on paper which most children love to do. It is rewarding to hold a crayon, move one's hand over the page and see bright red, green or yellow marks appear. As the child learns better coordinative control, parents can begin to create over-sized templates of letters and other shapes which the child can color in, copy or scribble over. Use plain, unlined paper for the preschool years. Create structure by whatever you choose to place on the paper, for example a picture or letter to be colored in or copied. Lined paper may make everything a bit more confusing, probably because the marks are distracting.

Do not fall into the trap of thinking that writing must be precise or that all the letters have to line up just right. Children are natural word processors and tend to "wrap" their sentences or words as they run out of space. Names printed like the following are OK.

                                                                    J I
M   G   A   RD   N   E   R

Initially, they can be of whatever color, shape, or size (like people) and placed just about anywhere on the page. Gradually, of course, the child will tighten up the letters, use less room and print his letters with more precision. No hurry here, of course. Just provide the mater-ials, sketch out what you want copied or colored, and enjoy the time with your child.

There are some who feel that reading is best taught by introducing writing first. In England many teachers promote this method in pre-school. The idea is to try and write down many, though not all, of the child's utterances. If the child says Simba and Pride Rock, the parent writes down Simba on one paper and Pride Rock on another. She tells the child that these are the words he just said and this is what they look like in writing. You can go on to draw pictures of Simba, tell stories, write more letters and words, or do whatever you want to.

AWARENESS

Item 45. Awareness of Self—body image (circle one)

Date of 1st rating _____ 2nd rating _____ 3rd rating _____

1. Shows no awareness of own body; does not know his nose or toes, for example.

2. Shows rudimentary and developing awareness in that he can point to some parts of his body.

3. Can point to all major parts of his body when they are named by parent.

4. Can point to and name all body parts; is clearly aware that his body parts are not those of someone else; recognizes self in mirror; knows own name.

5. Is clearly aware of own body parts, movements (touch your hand to your ear), and the fact that he is a separate entity from others.

What body image is and how to define it is a controversial topic among psychologists. For practical purposes, most of us carry an image in our mind about ourselves. My body will be ready for the beach this summer if I lose five pounds right now, for example. The individual's body image consists of his perception and awareness of the parts of his body as they function as a whole, including how he thinks he looks. Body image differs from body awareness. The latter involves both proprioceptive and kinesthetic feedback which help us become aware of and remain aware of where our body parts are and what they are doing. Body image, on the other hand, has to do with our perception of how we think we look and how we feel about ourselves.

Even though body awareness and body image are, conceptually at least, somewhat different, body image is primarily developed through body awareness. To assist the child in developing body awareness we play games such as "I'll pinch your nose" or "I'll bite your toes" or "This little piggy goes to market" and similar activities which, whether by original design or not, help teach the child about his body. Activities such as measuring oneself against a giant ruler on the back of the bedroom door or the wall of the child's room, mirror games, body tracing games in snow, sand, or a large piece of butcher block paper are useful. These activities help her begin to think of herself as a whole person, as an independent entity—a *self*.

Awareness of others and general social sensitivity will be covered in Chapter 10 which deals with the child's social-emotional development.

Item 46. Awareness of Cause–Effect Relationships (circle one)

Date of 1st rating _____2nd rating _____3rd rating _____

1. None apparent.

2. Some rudimentary understanding appears to be present, the child realizes, for example, when one tips a glass of water, it causes things to get wet.

3. Appears to have a good basic understanding with respect to such processes.

4. Is beginning to more clearly perceive cause-effect actions and can verbalize them fairly well.

5. Perceives basic cause-effect relations very clearly and can verbalize them.

Cause-effect relationships are often unclear, even for adults. Certainly, cause-effect for a child is an obscure bit of business. A child may think, for example, that umbrellas "cause" rain since he sees so many umbrellas when it is raining. In general, adults tend to use both scientific or empirical thinking in some matters and more superstitious or belief-grounded thinking in other areas. The engineer who may be coolly rational on the job may consult astrology charts about making personal decisions in her love life. Preschool-age children are not very rational; they indulge in magical thinking, and exist in their own world wherein fact and fantasy are easily confused. Systematic cause-effect thinking is unknown or barely present at this age. It will actually not be until the five to seven shift (see Chapter 11) that the young child will begin to move toward greater facility in the perception of cause-effect relations.

In any case, if the child is to begin to make sense out of the various correlated and uncorrelated events of his world, it is vital that he develop some basic understanding for and appreciation of cause-effect thinking. As stated, this will not come into bloom at all during the preschool years, but it is during these years that the groundwork is laid for good, critical, cause-effect understanding which will be useful in later childhood and adolescence. It is the lucky child who has some patient guide help him as he takes the first tentative steps into the morass of interconnected and unconnected events of daily life.

I once observed a gifted parent-teacher and a group of three year olds discuss "The Causes of Everything." The parent-teacher, using direct thinking out loud, questions (*Why* did it happen?), and references to hands-on projects in which the group members had participated led the children toward some initial understanding that some things cause other things to happen, some things do not cause events to happen though we sometimes think they do, and sometimes we don't know. She demonstrated that folding a paper plane's wing in a certain way *caused* the plane to veer left. She discussed how hitting a peer *caused* anger and, often, retaliation. She reminded the children of how their earth dam in the play yard *caused* water to back up and flow down a path constructed just for that purpose.

PROBLEM SOLVING

Although this chapter has focused on the development of memory, language and other basic cognitive skills, these abilities, as they develop and grow, become intertwined with another powerful human talent—problem solving. Despite the importance of problem solving (books have been devoted to just this subject), in the interest of space we will illustrate the basic concept with only one item here, albeit a lengthy one, in order to present the general idea.

Item 47. Problem Solving (circle one)

Date of 1st rating _____ 2nd rating _____ 3rd rating _____

1. Never attempts to figure out things such as how to open a door, close a box; tends to be passive and wait for someone else to solve the problem.

2. Rarely attempts to solve any sort of problem (finding a toy; putting on own clothes); tends to look to others for help.

3. Attempts to solve some problems/puzzles/toys by himself but tends to give up easily; shows no real trial-and-error approach to problems.

4. Attempts to solve most problems/puzzles, toys/life situations by himself; may request assistance at times but usually shows good perseverance and a trial-and-error attitude.

5. Attempts to solve almost any problem by himself; tends to be determined and confident; sticks with a problem and shows a good trial-and-error approach.

Here problem solving is viewed in its broadest sense. Children face "problems" which must be solved every day of their lives. How they go about dealing with these problems, their general success or failure in terms of "problem solving," begins to shape the nature of how they operate as older children to solve important academic and social problems. The latter subject, social problem solving, will be discussed in a later chapter, as well.

The ability to problem solve, though not a uniquely human trait, reaches its highest form in the human species. Virtually every aspect of life requires problem-solving ability of one kind or another. An individual can be good at solving problems in one area, academics let's say, but quite a bumbler in something else, working with his hands, for example. There is, however, some evidence that a type of *generalized problem-solving attitude* can be taught, a broad-based kind of problem solving approach which would be useful under almost any conditions. Some aspects of the generalized problem-solving attitude involve:

- Trial and error or almost random behavior as the individual begins to size up and "fool around with" the situation; the individual begins to sift and sort bits and pieces of the problem, to sort the pieces and begin to tentatively put them into place (part-whole relations; analysis and synthesis). These "pieces" may exist as thoughts, ideas or primitive hypotheses or they may literally exist as in jigsaw puzzles, model parts to be put together or toys that need to be repaired.

- The ability to tolerate frustration, to remain calm, thoughtful and rational under ambiguous or intially non-rewarding circumstances.

- The ability to delay gratification, to postpone the dictates of the pleasure principle—as in I want what I want when I want it, and I want it right now! We are told that Alexander the Great lost his temper when trying to solve the Gordian's knot, finally slashing it asunder with his sword. He thus "solved" the problem, while demonstrating no patience and no real capacity to think the situation through, and went on to rule the world. However, most of us must solve the problems of daily life in more standard ways.

- Novel responses are often required in effective problem solving so the ability to break out of a prelearned routine or preconceived manner of thinking to try something new is very useful.

- Patience

- Confidence in one's own thinking and doing skills; a belief in one's abilities.

How do we help our child develop a good attitude about solving problems?

First, we teach the child to be able to perceive and label various situations as "problems to be solved" as opposed to difficult or frustrating situations. If we reinforce the latter perception, he might respond by giving up, asking for help, or just "going blank" and not being able to think. Parents also play a large role as examples of how to act under the possible stressful problem situations. The parent may also act as a guide or prompter in assisting the child toward the development of good problem-solving responses.

Second, parents might want to use the "thinking-out-loud" technique which has been frequently mentioned in this book. This is an externalization of our adult inner logic or problem solving thinking. The child receives the benefit of hearing us mull over the problem and what we are planning to do about it. Thinking out loud is, of course, a form of vicarious trial and error. When the parent sits before a puzzling toy or construction kit and ponders out loud the probable best way to go about things before taking any action, the parent is demonstrating a cool, rational, and in-control problem solving method for the child to follow. When the child has seen you thinking like this before tackling a problem, it becomes easier for him to do the same.

Third, and embedded in the two points above, is the concept of gentle reinforcement of the child's efforts along with praise and attention for using good problem-solving techniques.

NOTES

1. Patterson, Gerald. *Living With Children: new methods for parents and teachers*. Champaigne (Ill.): Research Press. 1979.
2. Trelease, Jim. *The Read Aloud Handbook*. New York: Penguin. 1985. p. 62.

——10——
The Foundations of Creativity and Aesthetic Pleasure

My discussion now turns to creativity and aesthetic pleasure. This section is quite basic. Its purpose is to remind parents that creativity and aesthetic pleasures must start somewhere and are amenable to training and development.

On a personal level, I could probably, through much study and practice, become fairly knowledgeable about wine and food, although I do not feel it possible that I could ever become one of the great wine experts or chefs. My talents would reach a limit fairly quickly. The question is, though, would my appreciation of life be altered for the better? Probably. When I was young if someone had led me toward some special talent, perhaps in cooking or music or art, my overall skill level in the area of focus would almost certainly be heightened. And my overall enjoyment of life would have been expanded.

Multi-talented people are all around us. Some play lovely sonatas on the piano while, in their "real" vocation they run a business; others amaze us with their grace in ballroom dance and even win prizes, though they are doctors or lawyers by profession, and so on.

As mentioned, multi-talented people had to start somewhere. They were not just born with fully developed abilities. Each talent resides within us early in life. It will either develop or lie dormant, depending on the stimulation a child receives or does not receive in early childhood and beyond. Perhaps I shouldn't have resisted so strongly when my mother wanted me to take dancing lessons. My younger brother did not resist such lessons, became a terrific dancer, and to this day enriches his life with appearances as a dancer in various summer stock productions.

Parents need to provide a smorgasbord of early artistic and creative experiences for their children. Children will also find their own creative outlets when they are exposed to books, trips, camps, toys and so on. Our children cannot learn the pleasure and delights of Lincoln Logs or Legos if there are no such toys in their environment. They cannot learn about combining colors if they have no paint. They will not dance to music unless music is around them in their daily lives. Being introduced to music in school is not likely to make half the impact as a home where children are encouraged to listen to music and can hear family members playing instruments and enjoying the melodies.

Sensory appreciation involving taste, smell and touch are rarely taught in any formal way except, perhaps, in chef's school or a cabinetry refinishing class when we are already adults. Children, however, can be encouraged to explore these senses in what is called "incidental learning" as in "Doesn't that turkey cooking smell good!" "I love the smell of coffee." "The lemon is as bitter as sugar is sweet." "Feel how rough the sandpaper is." "This stone is so shiny and smooth."

The premise of this book, as we have said, is to help your child develop all of his potentials to as great a degree as possible consistent with good child rearing practices. Again, we are not trying to turn parents into taskmasters, scorekeepers, or grade givers. We are attempting to heighten parental awareness about the potential stored within their child and suggesting ways in which to help the child maximize that stored potential.

So, when we discuss taste, touch and smell it is not because we feel that the enhancement of these senses will make the child necessarily score higher on an IQ test or obtain better grades years later. Rather, I am saying that the development of all the child's senses and talents is likely to not only create a more efficient and well-integrated brain but, also, the child's quality of life will be enhanced as she becomes aware of the myriad aspects of life.

Let's turn now to a few areas involving creativity and/or aesthetic pleasure which appear to be "enhanceable" through parental involvement. Most parents will be able to think of many more activities and areas for enhancement.

Item 48. Response to Music (circle one)

Date of 1st rating _____ 2nd rating _____ 3rd rating _____

1. No apparent response.

2. Claps hands; moves to music holding hands with adult.

3. Taps or claps and moves to music with or without adult assistance.

4. Moves whole body in time with music; recognizes familiar songs.

5. Moves gracefully and in time with music; sings along on familiar songs or sings alone.

Most children respond in a natural and spontaneous manner to music. Even the infant seems to get pleasure by beating on something with a spoon or stick. Children quickly enjoy the songs from *The Little Mermaid, The Lion King,* and other tapes and videos as well as songs such as *Old McDonald Had A Farm, Now I Say My ABCs* and countless other nursery rhymes and lullabies. Later, after much familiarity with the basic rhythms and words, the child may make his own sounds. In our day and age, it is easy for parents to provide a wide assortment of music. Through tape cassettes and video we can fill the child's room, indeed, the whole house with music.

However, while simply filling the air with music is a move in the right direction, there are a few more steps the involved parent might consider. The parent who sings along with the music, twirling around or dancing with the child from time to time, adds another dimension. The parent's enjoyment of the music rubs off, the child picks up the rhythm and the words quickly, the child's speaking (singing) vocabulary expands as does the conceptual grasp (Who, after all, is coming around the mountain, driving six white horses?; the sing-song ABCs gradually becomes the familiar old ABCs, and so on).

After basic training with music, songs and rhymes in the home, it is easy for the parent to extend these activities into other areas. Consider the child who is along on a car ride. He is strapped in, usually in the rear seat of the car, and can see very little of the passing world. Most children sensibly fall asleep under these conditions. However, if the child is alert, use this travel time to play music and sing. Using a tape or CD player, you and your child can continue your

singing and general enjoyment of music as you roll down the high-
way.

Item 49. Response to Drawing/Painting Materials (circle one)

Date of 1st rating ———— 2nd rating ———— 3rd rating ————

1. No response. Does not use or have much apparent understanding of such materials.

2. Seems to enjoy employing a scribbling method as with crayons
   or creates messy dabbles of paint.

3. Uses crayons, pencils, paints, enjoys the activity but doesn't create much form.

4. Uses crayons, pencils, paints, enjoys the activity and can create
   basic shapes or "pictures" of something (though you might not
   recognize it until the child tells you what it is).

5. Uses these materials reasonably well and enjoys drawing, coloring or painting.

As with music, the child cannot develop an appreciation or a
skill in using art material unless such material is provided. At a
minimum, you will need to invest in crayons and paper. A more
expansive inventory might include an easel and paints, perhaps
a little work table or desk. Even when the basic materials are provided, you will still need to show the child how to use and enjoy
them

Remember, don't worry about whether the child is coloring
between lines or holding the crayon "correctly." Above all, don't
use what should be a fun time to start lecturing the child in "strict
teacher" fashion. You will probably turn your child off to any artistic
endeavor and you may also kill his desire to engage in further activities with you.

Be carefree and informal. Draw things yourself. Talk about it.
Encourage the child to draw, paint and talk about it. Set aside
some time each day for this kind of activity. This means keeping the
TV set off, of course, and continuing to help the child learn to enter-
tain himself through art and music and with picture books and
stories.

There are many excellent programs to promote the development
of your child's musical and artistic talents. These are usually available
or can be ordered through your local bookstore. For example, a

book which might be useful is Susan Ludington-Hoe's *How To Have A Smarter Baby: The Infant Stimulation Program for Enhancing Your Baby's Natural Development.* Another is Raelynn and Rachel Rein's, *How To Develop Your Child's Gifts and Talents During the Elementary Years.*

11

The Foundations of Social-Emotional Development

The young child's social and emotional development is inextricably linked with her physical and cognitive development. The fearful or anti-social child will be less likely to have as many experiences and positive interactions with peers and adults as will the outgoing, secure, socially competent child. We are aware that children, because of their different personalities, have various ways of responding to the world around them.

Some children have a very placid nervous system. They are not easily upset or startled. They have a calm disposition. Other children are much more reactive, even hyper-reactive. They tend to startle more easily and may be somewhat "clingy" or anxious. Some children react to new situations quite well, others have difficulty with new people or places; separating from a parent may be easier for some, harder for others. In this section, we talk of the child's overall attitude toward self and the world, cooperation with peers and others, response to adult suggestions and so on.

Although there are limitations, of course, to how much parents or other adults can change the basic personality of a child, there is no question that some of what we do or do not do as parents influences the development of the child's social skills and ultimately his behavior and attitude toward others. Children with good social skills are

119

generally liked by others. There are some children, however, who antagonize those around them.

A child who is pushy, won't share, shoves other children around, won't follow adult directions, whines, has tantrums, interrupts, is demanding of time and attention and so on is an unfortunate child. Eventually, he is not going to be well-liked by peers and even his preschool or elementary school teachers may begin to react negatively to him. At some point, these social difficulties become emotional problems. It behooves parents to consider gentle but consistent social training of their children.

Throughout this book we have been discussing cognitive enrichment or intellectual training as well as basic coordinative training. Clearly, some improvement can be made in these areas. We feel the same way about social training. Something can and should be done in this area, particularly if your child generally seems to have a poor attitude.

Item 51. General Attitude (circle one)

Date of 1st rating _____ 2nd rating _____ 3rd rating _____

1. Insecure, fearful and/or seemingly unhappy much of the time.

2. Timid, rather dependent on parent for security.

3. Varies from timid and inhibited to appropriate participation in activities with peers.

4. Varies in apparent degree of security or insecurity, largely depending on the situation.

5. Almost always spontaneous, open, and willing to participate in activities with peers or adults.

Parents do their child a great favor when they insist that she exhibit appropriate social behavior. It would be very desirable, also, if we could teach our children to view life in a relatively calm, open, friendly way. Although it may not be possible to teach some children how to have a sunny disposition and to enjoy life, there is certainly no harm in trying. Indeed, it's wise to make an attempt since the outcome can only be positive. In fact, the "likability quotient" and the attitude of a person may be as important in life as his IQ. As we have taken the position that intelligence can be enhanced with help from parents, we feel that a child's "likability" can also be enhanced with his parent's help.

It is obvious that children are not born knowing how to act in social situations. We all must learn, usually fairly early in life, how to treat others in a decent manner, how to share, take turns and wait in line, for example. Although some of us are born with naturally pleasant and kind dispositions that cause others to consider us "likable," many of us need a good deal of coaching in this area. And, as we grow up we may need a fair amount of more or less continuous socialization training. We need to learn not only how to act but also how to show a reasonably good attitude toward our siblings, peers, teachers and parents.

The good parent will use benign, but firm, coaching or discussion when her child uses negative or inappropriate behavior or manifests a sulky, negative attitude. She will also try to pay attention to the child's positive behaviors and attitudes and praise this type of conduct, thus encouraging the child to continue to act in this manner. If necessary, the good parent will redirect the child and walk him through certain scenes again. She might instruct the grumpy, scowling child to sit down or leave the room until he can come in with a smile on his face.

Parents must confront the child about his negative behavior, they should label the behavior ("You are acting in a very *rude* way right now") without labeling the child. They must describe with words or through role playing the exact behavior they expect to see ("I want to see a big smile on that handsome face."). Remember to be very distinct and definite in your teaching of the magic words all children need to know and use, "Please" and "Thank you."

Confront negative behavior instantly. Be an "in-your-face" parent in a loving but firm way. Label behavior for what it is, selfish or mean, for instance. Indicate what behavior you want the child to show under the circumstances at this moment. Again, reinforce the child with praise and attention for using the new and more positive behavior.

Remember, too, that human behavior is very complex. It is unlikely that your child will need only one "lesson" to develop pro-social behavior and reduce anti-social behavior. Prepare yourself to repeat these lessons. All the while, be very supportive. You will be glad you did. And, ultimately, so will your child.

Item 52. Sense of Humor (circle one)

Date of 1st rating _____ 2nd rating _____ 3rd rating _____

1. Too young to assess.

2. Laughs and giggles at dolls, peek-a-boo games, seems to enjoy people.

3. Old enough and alert enough to "get" the humor in some situations such as certain videos or stories.

4. Can usually get the humor in a video, story or interaction between self and another.

5. Generally is quick to perceive humor; picks up nuances well in conversation, videos, TV, stories.

A sense of humor is a great help in this world. The ability to be able to see the funny side of things can make a difference between bouncing back from bad luck and moving forward in life or slipping into a "woe is me" debilitating discouragement or a depression. Although I once accepted the idea that one either did or did not have a natural sense of humor, I now believe that one's "sense of humor" can be enhanced and sharpened. It is helpful to the child, of course, if he has a parent who possesses a good sense of humor or, at least, can appreciate the value of humor. We're not referring to joke-telling here, though jokes, puns, and the like have their place. this section discusses the general ability of an individual to perceive the wry, ironic or very funny side of various events or situations.

It appears that almost all children have a "humor capacity" and, with training, this capacity can be developed. Freud saw humor as a great asset and felt that, "Humor can...be conceived as the loftiest of the defense functions (coping mechanisms)."[1] If strength and skill and mental quickness are "good things" for the child, then we must also see the value of a major coping skill such as humor. The world is a hard place and, as M. Scott Peck has succinctly noted in his book, *A Road Less Traveled*, "life is difficult."[2] Humor, then, is a useful tool in daily life.

Our efforts to instill a sense of humor, however, should not start at too high or too abstract a level. We would not expect preschool age children, for example, to understand the humor in a character such as Falstaff, or the dry humor of Mark Twain or even simple jokes or puns. The development of humor in young children may start with basic discriminations in pictures and stories wherein the question asked is, essentially, "What is funny about that?" The Stanford-Binet IQ test has a section in which the young child is shown pictures of various incongruous situations such as mice and a cat hanging out together. The child is then asked to state what he thinks is funny about each picture. It is clear, then, that Lewis Terman and the other creators of this famous intelligence test considered humor to be an integral part of intelligence. Thus, humor is an important aspect in terms of our ability to size up and grasp the content of situations. We do well to help the child develop this sense.

But where do find material for the preschooler? First, the local educational supply can help. We can use picture books such as the *Where's Waldo?* series and books by Dr Seuss such as *The Cat In the Hat* as we read and talk with the child about the antics of Thing 1 and Thing 2 and how the cat, at the end, noting that he "Always picks up all his playthings" comes in with a funny machine and gets the house spic and span again before mother arrives home. Through the years children have laughed as Pinochio's nose grows longer when he tells a lie, also delighting in the little bird's nest that the Disney artist placed on the end of his long nose after he had told a series of fibs. But, the younger children, especially, laugh *after* it has been pointed out that the nose was a strange place for a bird's nest, imagine one on your nose, and so on.

Secondarily, however, we fall back on our resources. Each parent has to think about the funny or humorous incidents in his daily life and share these with the child in a way that he can understand.

To work on the enhancement of humor, then, the parent has to be quite pro-active and use many resources. In addition to books, games, videos, photos and daily incidents, you can draw on memories. For example, you can say, "Can you remember the funniest story you ever heard?" Or, "Do you remember that funny clown at the circus?" As stated, it helps to have a great sense of humor. If you don't feel that your own sense of humor is adequate, but you perceive the desirability of helping to develop humor in your child, then using the techniques mentioned here will probably help loosen you up, too. You and your child will then have twice as much fun together.

Item 53. Response to New Social Situations (circle one)

Date of 1st rating _____ 2nd rating _____ 3rd rating _____

1. Unable to cope; may be fearful; clings to parent; does not explore.

2. Handles new situations only marginally well and usually only with much adult support.

3. Can sometimes cope on his own though needs initial adult support and urging.

4. Can usually cope on his own though tends to need initial adult support or urging.

5. Almost always copes well and adjusts to new situations without adult assistance.

In general, the child who is socially, intellectually and physically competent can and will handle most new social situations well. The younger child, of course, has had a shorter "training time" for dealing with new, complex or confusing social situations. Therefore, some children will understandably enter such situations reluctantly and often only with some adult coaching. For example, "Go over there and play with Billy on the sliding board. He looks like he's having a lot of fun."

The development of the Mommy and Me and Gymboree type programs appears to be useful to the modern child and her parents. These programs probably do more to help the parents work on their parenting skills than they do for the children's development directly. Socialization training for the young child also takes place informally through the parent's personal contacts. Mother may meet friends in the neighborhood park or in a home and socialize while her children play with other kids. Additional social skill development occurs for all children, of course, when they enter preschool and, then, kindergarten and elementary school.

Parents need to expose their children to a variety of social situations with same age peers and with other children of varying ages. If children have few interactions with other children, for whatever the reason, they tend not to develop smooth social skills. This makes sense, of course, when we consider that "social skills" are, by definition, learned skills applied in various social situations.

The naturally outgoing, gregarious child will need little extra assistance to develop his social skills. He enjoys being with others, whether peers or adults, and generally tends to get along very well. Also, children who can separate from parents easily and interact well with others are, for the most part, secure children who have formed solid love relationships at home. Family relationships are, of course, the foundation on which people build other relationships.

Since some children are, by nature or disposition, less outgoing than others they may need special attention to improve their social skill development. Children who have had inconsistent parenting during the early years may also require more help. The "naturally" shy child will also have difficulty with new or strange situations. In either case, the child needs increasing "doses" of exposure to peers in small play groups. Again, the commercial baby classes can be useful too, as can informal contacts with other parents of young children so that the children can learn to mingle and play together.

The parent must be careful not to pressure or push the fearful or shy child. We can discuss the child's fears with him to some extent, and help him with his feelings. We can tell him that these feelings are normal and natural, and urge him gently to override the feelings of shyness and try some new situations. A positive message should be embedded in your words. For example, "As you feel more and more sure of yourself and happy with your new friends, you will be wanting to play with them more often, and you will enjoy this a lot."

When you talk to your child he can understand the tone if not the words in their entirety. Your words should evoke warm emotional support of him at all times. The child also needs to trust you and what you say. Don't tell him something you know to be wrong. He won't, for example, necessarily enjoy the waterslide the first time out. As with many things in life, he may need much splashing around in the shallow end of the pool before he tries the deep water.

Sometimes a parent's attitude can hinder a shy or fearful child's social development. We have noted that the parent should not push or pressure the child into new situations when the child is afraid. If you are my guide on a strange mountain trail and you suddenly leave me, calling out that being on my own will be good for me, I might survive but I sure won't trust you or even want to be with you in the future. If you pressure a child you are not going to gain his trust and he may even become angry or withdrawn.

As parents we need to make sure our own fears about new situations don't seep down to the child. Parents of shy or fearful children often become uptight in advance as they anticipate all the problems and possible embarrassment their child's behavior will cause. You must not be ruled by fear of what others think; be governed, rather, by what you think is best for you and your child. If you feel that you should hang around on the playground or in the classroom for a while, then do so. You and the child will generally know when this is no longer necessary. When in doubt, ask an experienced parent or teacher whom you trust to provide some advice to you on this matter.

One last point here has to do with the value of stories. Stories which the shy child can relate to can be very useful. All children, in fact, need to hear and see stories of little ones who gradually grow up or change in some way to become more competent and accepted. "The Ugly Duckling" is a powerful story that most of us identify with at some level. Children need to be exposed to stories to which they can relate and which will help them see that although they are small and shy now, they will be different in the future.

Item 54. Response to Adult Direction (circle one)

Date of 1st rating _____ 2nd rating _____ 3rd rating _____

1. No apparent understanding of directions and/or willingness to follow.

2. Tends to be openly negative and/or evasive.

3. Reluctantly cooperative.

4. Usually cooperative, may argue or protest a bit in a "normal" or usual manner.

5. Generally cooperative, open, and willing; very little protest over most requests.

We tend to assume that a preschool age child who appears to be developmentally and psychologically normal can hear and understand what we say to him. Consequently, when the child does not follow directions well, we may label him as headstrong or willful. This may or may not be the case; thus, it is wise to do a little checking with respect to hearing, auditory memory and auditory processing.

Your pediatrician can check the child's hearing or you can do so yourself using a simple "whisper test." Although not precise, the whisper test will give you some idea of the child's hearing ability. All you do is stand behind the child and recite numbers or letters, asking him to hold up a hand when he first hears you and tell you what number or letter he first hears. Start low and whisper more and more loudly. If you feel that there is no problem, you can conclude that the child is probably hearing your directions but not following them for some other reason. You may want to review the previous section on auditory processing and auditory memory at this time.

The point here is that you, initially, should not just assume that your child is being negative and simply not doing what you ask. He may, as stated, just not hear very well or he may have a developmental immaturity in areas involving auditory memory or auditory processing and decoding. If you feel that your child may have a problem in any one of these areas, professional consultation should be sought starting with your pediatrician and possibly extending to developmental testing by a speech and hearing specialist.

If you think that your child can hear normally, but he isn't understanding you, check your own directions to ascertain if you are possibly using phrases that may be too abstract or too general. Phrases such as "Be good" or "Act like a nice boy" are quite abstract and imprecise to him. With little ones, especially those who aren't picking up quickly on abstract terms, describe exactly what it is you want the child to do ("I want you to put down your crayons. Come over here to the table. Sit down and eat your lunch.").

Since children are going to be difficult or negative some portion of the time, the parent must give some careful thought to how to handle this behavior.

To develop a child's sense of cooperation and self-discipline, the parent must be in control of herself. The parent who has little self-discipline, who flies into a rage and tantrums, yells or hits helps promote a child's anger and fear and, later, avoidance. The parent who is calm and consistently insists on certain reasonable behaviors will help the child develop solid inner controls and strong self-discipline.

But, even if we do the best we can to instill self-control in our child there will be times when he exhibits negative behavior. If you are calm and consistent, you may either 1) override the child's protests and gently guide her toward what you desire her to do or 2) cut the child some slack with a courteous if-then or when-then contingency statement such as, "When you finish the picture, then come get your lunch." Follow this with another *then*, "Then we will read or take a walk."

Do not reinforce a child's negative or inappropriate behavior. If you give into negative outbursts and tantrums, *especially* every now and then, you have placed the child on an intermittent schedule of reinforcement. An intermittent schedule is like a gambling schedule, every once in awhile you win. The child learns to go into a tantrum or manipulation mode when he wants something, even though you do not give in every time but only some of the time. Some of the time is good enough to build a very strong habit pattern.

Many older children are quite conscious of the fact that every now and then they get their way by arguing, begging or throwing a tantrum. Younger children are usually unconscious of why they go into tantrum or whine mode, but it's almost always because they sometimes get what they want by behaving in one of those ways.

In any case, you do yourself and your child a real favor by holding even, staying consistent and avoiding giving in to manipulative behavior. Realize that you will have to use reasonable if-then or when-then contingency statements fairly often. In the extreme case, use a modified time-out procedure and simply time yourself out. That is, withdraw your attention from the child (do not fight with him to put him in his room, for instance), just become less warm and a bit more aloof. Your message is that you are not going to focus on his needs for the time being. Do not extend your "self time out" too long. That is not fair. Do not overuse withdrawal of privileges or timing yourself out for unimportant transgressions since these methods will become less effective if you do.

The younger the child, the more gentle the teaching. Be consistent. Be clear. Be kind.

Item 55. Individual Play (circle one)

Date of 1st rating _____ 2nd rating _____ 3rd rating _____

1. Does not play alone.

2. Plays alone unwillingly; dependent upon adult participation or structure.

3. Occasionally will play alone in selected activities.

4. Can play alone but tends not to do so for very long periods.

5. Can play alone, enjoys it, can stay with independent activities for fairly long periods.

If you learn to like yourself and be your own best friend, you possess a resource which you can never lose. Additionally, we intuitively realize that creativity often flows from thoughts and feelings generated by individual work and/or contemplation. Poems, concertos, paintings, sculpture and books are rarely, if ever, created by committee. Creative minds often function well in solitude. To be quiet and to be alone one has had to develop inner discipline and habits of mind which allow one to be alone but not lonely.

We have mentioned several times the advent of the modern Mommy and Me classes and Gymboree which involve parents and their very young children. These programs are generally very good because they heighten parental awareness of the needs of the young child and help the child's development. They also provide early socialization experiences for the children under very benign and pleasant conditions But, as important as it is to learn to be with others in a good way, it is also critically important to learn how to be with yourself in a good way.

The point is, we must set conditions so that the child is not only provided with all the varying kinds of stimulation we have discussed throughout the book but, also, quiet or "down" time, as well. This does not, of course, include watching TV. Some children adapt well and quickly to being left alone to putter around or play as they wish. However, until the child is old enough to be capable of longer periods of coloring, drawing or playing with puzzles, blocks or other toys the parent is usually the most fun plaything in the child's world. Initially, she helps the child learn how to play alone, for playing alone, too, is a learned activity.

At the start of teaching how to play alone, the parent plays with the child. This is how you would start regardless of whether your child is a "young" preschooler or older. You might build with blocks, play with the Fisher-Price "little people," draw, use coloring books, read or do other pleasant activities. When the child is happily engaged in the activity, you move yourself out of the play situation for a very brief period of time. Less time, say, than it takes to fix a cup of instant coffee. Then, come back into the activity with the child.

As the child begins to enjoy the play for itself, not just because you're there, time yourself out of the activity for a bit longer. Perhaps as long as it takes to sip your coffee and glance at the front page of the newspaper. This type of teaching is called "fading." You are literally generating an activity with your child then fading yourself out gradually. Eventually, the child will (if you do this well) be able to play for longer and longer periods alone.

Some educators advocate the cold turkey approach. They recommend turning off the TV, providing some toys, and letting the child develop his own fun activities. Perhaps you would prefer to use your own method that reflects something between the fading and the cold turkey approaches.

There is no set rule for judging how much individual play is too much or too little. Some children will play alone more readily and for longer periods of time than others. Some are natural loners, others are more people oriented. I would become concerned if the child plays almost exclusively by himself and either cannot or will not interact with peers or adults other than parents. On the other hand, the child who never plays alone may be overly dependent upon others for stimulation or structure and not yet have developed "play alone" skills. As with most things in our lives and with our children, as well, balance is desired. Thus, the child needs to develop the ability to play alone at times and with others at other times. In our modern, hurried life, however, play-alone skills may be overlooked by many teachers and parents. The point here is that playing alone skills are:

- important for a child to possess,

- not pathological, and

- the foundation stones of creativity and imagination.

NOTES

1. Freud, Sigmund. *Wit and Its Relation to the Unconscious.* New York: Modern Library, 1938. p. 801.
2. Peck, M. Scott. *The Road Less Traveled.* New York: Simon & Schuster, 1978, p. 15.

III

THE SECOND FIVE YEARS

12

The Five to Seven Year Shift

The previous section focused on what might be considered the basic building blocks of higher level thinking—receptive and expressive language skills, visual and auditory perception, the ability to attend and concentrate, memory functions, basic coordination, self esteem and social skills. Following the tremendous expansion of cognitive capacity in the early years there are two more known shifts in brain functioning. The first begins at about age five and is completed at about age seven; the second begins at approximately the beginning of puberty and continues until mid or late adolescence.

Part III will discuss the development of higher order thinking skills and how parents can help maximize them. These skills, in turn, will set the stage for the integration of new and more expanded cognitive capacities following the changes of puberty and early adolescence. But, for now, we'll briefly focus on that time in life, at about age five years, when the child begins to leave early childhood and move toward a different and more powerful thinking capacity. This time is known as the "five to seven shift."

According to Dr. Melvin Konner, an early childhood specialist at Harvard University, this change in the five to seven age range is largely biological. He states:

> Among other things [at this age], there is a stabilization of brain-wave rhythms...Children become capable of new kinds of learning, and mature grammar is attained in language development. These changes hint at fundamental growth in the brain at this age. Some experts point to the completion of myelination—the laying down of more rapidly conducting sheaths along the nerve paths. Others see changes in the

granule cells—tiny, densely packed cells of the hippocampus, a brain region crucial to memory.[1]

Additionally, at this age, the child begins to lose baby teeth while making considerable gains in height and weight.

Of course, in our culture the child at this age is also being weaned away from home or preschool to spend more time in the structured environment of kindergarten and the early grades. Thus, a higher level of cognitive stimulation is impacting the child at this time. On a daily basis and for many hours per day he is exposed to language, symbols, ideas, rules, order and organization. He will develop a greater awareness of time, interact more with peers, and be introduced to games and other activities.

About fifteen to twenty percent of our children will not be happy with the introduction of reading, writing (printing), spelling, and basic math skills. Approximately this percentage of children have underlying developmental immaturities or, more seriously, significant perceptual dysfunctions. Some three to five percent of children will manifest some degree of attention deficit disorder,[2] often with hyperactivity or some form of perceptual dysfunction as well. Many children will mature past or "outgrow" the developmental immaturities, though certain kinds of school work may be frustrating for awhile. However, if the child has deeper level perceptual dysfunctions, it is not likely that he will either outgrow them or be able to function well in school. Such children have learning differences or learning disabilities, depending on the term used at a particular school. The down side is that these children are likely to experience many frustrations in their academic work and, worst case scenario, develop negative self-esteem, low self-confidence, and a poor attitude toward school that could lead to a full-blown school phobia.

If a preschooler has developed to a point where he can legitimately be rated as a "5" in most or all areas of Section II, he will be unlikely to experience difficulty when he enters elementary school, since he would be judged "kindergarten ready" for most schools.

For the happy eighty five percent or so of children who manifest no learning problems, the years during and following the five to seven shift are, for the most part, more or less steady ones from a developmental standpoint. The child in this category is moving away from early childhood. She has learned how to separate from mother or father and look to her teacher as a kind of parent surrogate for many hours of the day. She socializes well and enjoys her peer interactions. She likes to learn and apply her new basic reading, writing and math skills. She begins to think more and more like an adult though much of her logic is still primitive.

Freud termed this time the "latency period," meaning that many of the child's feelings and developmental issues were steady, somewhat dormant or latent.[3] Piaget noted a time of the development of operational thought.[4] And schools, in this country at least, recognize the five-to-six year old period as being about right for the initiation of formal instruction.

As the child moves through this five to seven shift and on into the latency period, many developmental crises may transpire, with all affecting cognitive development and functioning to a more or less extent. Negative events such as death of a parent, divorce by parents, a frightening teacher or a school bully, not fitting in socially, being made to feel stupid academically (learning disorder or over-pressuring parent), sexual or physical abuse, natural disasters such as earthquakes or hurricanes, birth of a sibling, loss of a grandparent by death or friend by school transfer may undermine the child's cognitive functioning and school performance.

This is, of course, the stuff of life and all of us face some or several of these issues. And we all get through them one way or another. However, in the first decade of life, one has few coping mechanisms developed as yet. The child even has some difficulty "compartmentalizing," not yet having learned how to skillfully use this major defense mechanism. Adults compartmentalize all the time. We put our domestic problems aside, for example, so that we can function at work and not lose our jobs or be embarrassed by ineptitude. We tend to shut out, except for selected moments during the evening news, perhaps, most of the horrors of the world—the hunger and misery of others, crime and major disasters.

Children tend to use denial and distortion of reality a good deal. These defense mechanisms assist the child in warding off the terrors of their world. When these defenses are penetrated by some event too large for the child's immature ego structure to deal with, such as the 1994 earthquake in Los Angeles, the child (or adult) may become almost immobilized by fear and immune to attempts by others to reassure him. The very young child will ordinarily be too young to be overly affected by such events, or family problems; the middle childhood age child, following the five to seven shift, may be highly negatively impacted by such factors, however. These factors are beyond her control but no longer beyond her apprehension.

Problem solving, comprehension and learning, in general, are based on acquired knowledge. Children, as well as adults assimilate new information and process it on the basis of prior experience. Since the younger the child the less background he has available with which to process new information, the more incomplete the processing will be. The young child, then, must rely on primitive processing. The Beauty and Beast watch purchased by her parents at Disneyland the day before which shifts from showing Beauty to showing Beast depending on the angle with which it is held becomes confusing for the young child. She is not sure when she will see Beauty or when Beast may appear, and she is also not sure if either is real or not. Her best bet may be to bury it in her sand box, which is just what a young friend of mine did.

The mid-childhood individual, on the other hand, has moved through the five to seven shift and now thinks differently than she did before. She has much more background information, acquired by living a bit longer. Now she can compare and contrast aspects of reality. She is a thinking and an aware being. She is ready to begin absorbing more information about her world, to begin learning how to think about herself, others, and the world around her.

NOTES

1. Konner, Melvin. *Childhood*. Boston: Little, Brown. 1991. pp. 239–240.
2. *Diagnostic and Statistical Manual of Mental Disorders—Fourth Edition*. Washington, D.C.: American Psychiatric Association. 194. p. 82.
3. Freud, Sigmund. *The Basic Writings of Sigmund Freud*. New York: Random House, 1938. pp. 582–584.
4. Piaget, Jean. *Play, Dreams, and Imitation*. New York: Norton. 1962.

13

The Enhancement of Right Brain Thinking

The human brain is actually two brains, each capable of advanced mental functions. When the cerebrum is divided surgically, it is as if the cranium contained two separate spheres of consciousness.[1]

Dr Michael Gazzaniga, Brain Researcher

... we face so many simultaneous problems whose solutions depend upon our ability to grasp the relationship of parts to wholes ... split—and whole brain studies have led to a new conception of human knowledge, consciousness, and intelligence. All knowledge cannot be expressed in words, yet our education is based almost exclusively on its written or spoken forms ... But the artist, dancer, and mystic have learned to develop the nonverbal portion of intelligence.[2]

Dr Robert Ornstein, Brain Researcher

Our culture emphasizes left brain thinking. Our schools are well-suited for verbal, logical, linear type thinkers but are often not well-equipped to foster talents involving non-verbal, visual-spatial, perceptual-conceptual, or ability to perceive part-whole relations. Despite the presence of some music, art and drama classes most of our children's education in schools is focused on linear, logical, sequential, cause-effect type thinking. Schools may, at times, actually discourage or react negatively to more intuitive, non-verbal type thinking.

The concept of left brain and right brain difference is now more or less established, though not all aspects of the functioning of the separate hemispheres, whether acting in concert or separately, is yet known. Sally Springer and Georg Deutsch, in their book, *Left Brain, Right Brain*,[3] characterize the functions of the two brain hemispheres as follows:

Left Hemisphere	Right Hemisphere
Verbal	Nonverbal, visual-spatial
Sequential, temporal, digital	Simultaneous, spatial, analogical
Logical, analytical	Gestalt, synthetic
Rational	Intuitive
Western thought	Eastern thought

Another criticism often raised in discussions of what intelligence is and how it can be measured is that intelligence tests, like schools, measure primarily left brain functioning while more or less ignoring the talents of the right brain. The criticism that intelligence tests do not assess global cognitive functioning very well is not accurate with respect to all IQ tests. The Wechsler Intelligence Scale for Children— Third Edition (WISC-III), previously mentioned, does assess verbal and non-verbal functioning and arrives at a global assessment with a Full Scale IQ score. The psychologist is able to use the Verbal IQ, which is a good predictor of academic success, the Performance IQ, a good measure of non-verbal or right brain functioning, or the Full Scale IQ in order to size up how left and right brain functioning blends or where it doesn't, or if there are underlying perceptual problems.

Psychologists, educators and others who think about thinking are, as stated above, frequently chastised for being partial to the verbal areas of intelligence. But, since the non-verbal areas are critical to whole brain or maximal intellectual functioning, it seems fair that we start with some considerations of the enhancement of the non-verbal or right brain functions.

The activities suggested in this chapter and the next touch upon only a very limited number of training possibilities which you can use with your child. These are meant as illustrative; it is assumed that each parent will elaborate on and add to such activities based on her child's needs and interests. In any case, the activities involved in "brain training," as it were, are aimed at strengthening engrams or traces among the neurons and, through repeated exposure to all sorts of activities, stimulating the development of "neuronal nets" or networks within the child's brain.[4] In other words, new activities create new connections within the brain. These connections are reinforced and grow stronger and faster with repetition of the activity, whether it be thinking or doing. Some relevant areas for the enhancement of non-verbal cognitive skills are as follows:

DISCRIMINATION OF SUBTLE CUES

According to psychologist Dr Gary Groth-Marnat, the discrimination of subtle cues "…is a measure of visual concentration and is a non-verbal test of general information. It involves discovering consistency and inconsistency by paying close attention to the environment and accessing remote memory."[5] To perform well on a task involving seeing what is missing from a picture the child should have good reality contact, be able to discriminate subtle cues well and be able to perceive the difference between relevant and irrelevant cues.

Children who can do this well tend to be able to quickly and efficiently perceive fine details in their environments. In school, for example, they understand the directions or the small cues on bar graphs. They grasp that the teacher has said to do every odd numbered problem out of the first twenty problems and they do not come home complaining about having to do all twenty problems. They quickly recognize the visual information presented, whether in academic or social situations.

Children who discern fine details poorly tend to have difficulties in concentration and obvious problems in visual-perceptual functioning. This is not to say that there is a visual problem and the child needs eyeglasses, though this may be so and tests may be necessary. Rather, children who do not pick up on subtle cues have problems with directions at school, may miss the "sign" on math problems and subtract rather than add or vice versa and may have social problems since they do not pick up the nuances of certain social interactions readily, for instance, the arched eyebrow; or the fact that he is talking too much and others are becoming annoyed.

You can help the child develop in this area by showing him how to become more alert to small details and to things which are in some way out of synch within the picture. Basically, we are talking about good observational skills. The *Where's Waldo?* books come to mind. These books feature a very large number of people who are, say, at the beach. Among the many of people and other details in the picture will be Waldo. The task is to find him. There are many game books which contain puzzles or problems of this sort.

A good observational game that is in many of these types of books shows a picture of, say, a hunter in what appears to be Africa. There are road signs, a tiger attacking him, a servant running away. The hunter is ready to shoot his pistol at the tiger; he has a knife strapped to his belt; there is a jeep broken down in some bushes, and so on. Dozens of details. You are to look at the picture for one minute only. Then, you turn the page and try to see recall the details from the many questions that are asked about the scene. Was it a tiger or panther; a jeep or a truck? Did he have a canteen with him? How many towns were noted on the sign? A variation on this game has the hunter telling his story to someone. The story is full of errors. You turn the page and try to recall the errors after looking for one minute at this same scene with the hunter.

Many years ago my scoutmaster urged us to hone observational skills by looking for thirty seconds at store windows, then looking away and trying to write down every item which could be recalled. In the woods, we were to observe plants, animals, rock formations and so on and then write these down every ten minutes, thus creating, as he called it, an "observational journal."

Children's observation for detail is enhanced by someone merely calling attention to this as a skill, as the scoutmaster did, and as many hunters presumably have done when training their young people in the art of tracking. If observational acuity is emphasized as a skill, then exercise of this skill becomes more fun for the child.

Activities which are quite directly applicable to school involve preparing or preconditioning the child to observe material which you or she is about to read. Barbara Vitale, author of *Unicorns Are Real: a right brained approach to learning,* calls this technique "grounding."[6] Her little book is full of many excellent suggestions for development of right hemisphere efficiency. Using her grounding technique, which could also be called a priming technique, the parent and child look the book over and examine the pictures. The parent asks questions such as what is going on in the picture, what might be happening and what might happen next, how many colors do you see, how many people are in the picture, who might they be and so on.

For additional training, the parent might ask the child to find the first question mark on the page, the first name and so on. Care must be taken, of course, not to overdo all these questions before ever getting to the fun of the story. Through this method, the child has been given some practice in observing detail and has been primed to enjoy and understand the story better. After the story, if appropriate, you could browse the pictures again with your child relating little details to things you read in the story. Again, don't overdo it or you might ruin the fun of the story or the child's desire to read with you.

ARRANGING PICTURES IN SEQUENCES

The activity called "sequencing" has to do with how and why one set of events flows into another set of events and the ability to anticipate an event from a preceding event. Academically, the student must constantly discern how one thing flowed from another or "caused" an event to happen. Comic books or the funny papers in your newspaper are good examples of sequenced material. One frame relates to another frame in some kind of connected sequence. Cut up a sequence of comic book frames, then mix them up. Ask the child to put them in their right order so that they tell a sensible story.

Sequencing ability clearly also involves attention to detail. Some children cannot sequence very well, though their attention to detail may be quite good; sometimes vice versa. Both skills are useful to us academically and socially. In terms of sequencing, it is very necessary to be able to perceive that one event precedes another as well as how these events fit together in cause-effect manner. The girl waits at the bus stop. The bus comes and she gets on. She looks out the window as the bus pulls away.

This is elemental, but many children don't quickly process all this material and smooth it out in sequence. When they can't do this, there is likely to be much difficulty in comprehending a total situation and dealing with it. These children just do not seem to "get it" with respect to how and why other people, children and adults, do what they do when they do it. Academically, difficulties arise because of the lack of skill in perceiving how material or information flows together and how one event caused or preceded another.

Another helpful activity is to cut up a story into different segments, perhaps paragraph by paragraph, then have the child put them into an order that makes a sensible story. The child can also be asked to describe the events in a movie he has seen. How did it start, what happened then and how did it end. If the child has difficulty with a whole movie, start with shorter cartoons or videos or simply prompt the child yourself on parts he does not remember (assuming you have also seen the movie or video). This story telling technique can be based on almost any activity the child has been engaged in ranging from school, to birthday parties or sports. The child is more likely to be happy in this activity when the parent shows interest and encourages the child to remember the order of events.

PERCEPTUAL ORGANIZATION

The enhancement of perceptual organization or the ability to grasp the "big picture" conceptually is an important cognitive ability. Training in this activity depends upon both availability of certain materials as well as on a parent or other helper. Most young children are "naturals" at taking things apart, putting things together (more or less), and usually just like to play with blocks, play logs, Legos and other manipulables. Fancy material is actually not really required, though beautifully made wooden and plastic toys abound. But pots and pans, egg cartons, any kind of boxes which can be stacked can be used, too. Sand play and creating constructions in sand is another activity which is useful. There are also games involving the continual adding of a block to a stack until the stack falls down (the player who places the block that causes the fall is the "loser" of that round). This is useful, fun and a high participatory activity for a parent to engage in with her child.

ABC block sets with the alphabet, numbers and pictures on different sides are helpful here. To be most effective, of course, the parent and child should play with these materials often in an easy and pleasant manner. The parent should use the thinking out loud verbalizations which we have previously discussed. For instance, while she plays with the blocks she can say, "Let's put the A here, then a B on top of it, now let's find a C and put on top of that." Or, "Let's build a *room. First,* I'll put a block *down* here for the *base.* The base will be *under* the other blocks. Then, you *add* one on top of that. How *high* shall we make it? *Three* blocks tall? *Four*?" Parents will quickly perceive the potential for conceptual expansion (first, block, base) as well as prepositional or general vocabulary development and matching number words (three, four) to actual numbers of blocks used. Also, middle and upper elementary school age children can benefit from playing board games such as Battleship because this helps in developing skills involving spatial relationships and orientation in space.

This kind of teaching and learning takes place informally and often in most families, though usually not in as thought out a manner as is being outlined here.

Any kind of activity which involves moving or placing or replacing objects in various configurations will work to enhance perceptual/conceptual organization. Building model cars or planes or bird houses, fitting Play-do forms together; playing with shapes and twisting and turning spatial representations on a computer; folding paper to create airplanes and hats; and simply playing around with blocks that must be constructed to make them look like a design are all activities which go toward helping develop skills in perceptual organization.

Organizing physical space is a useful tool to enhance the development of general perceptual organization. Cleaning up a room or a garage and organizing material and space is a good activity though, with most children, considerable assistance is initially necessary. If organizing one's desk or room is regarded as a fun activity, especially when done with mom or dad's help, general organizational skills can be enhanced.

Children with poor or undeveloped perceptual-spatial skills would understandably shy away from organizing a room or desk since this would be difficult for them. These children probably need the most help in this area, though they may be so resistant that it is hard to engage them. Usually, if the parent will help, the children will perform the activity. The parent should, of course, involve the child in the planning phase by asking where the child thinks certain items should be put or stored and, also, using the thinking aloud technique, for example, "I wonder how it would look if we put the desk over against that wall? Perhaps it would make the room look larger and give you more room to walk."

PART-WHOLE RELATIONSHIPS

The obvious activity for enhancement of this domain of intelligence that embodies the perception of part-whole relations, use of cues, and spatial relations is jigsaw type puzzles. These puzzles come in varying degrees of difficulty and it is very easy to find puzzles which fit your child's age and developmental level.

At a broader level, an approach which will perhaps better illustrate the relationship between skill in jigsaw puzzles and dealing with part-whole relations, is to engage in a left brained activity such as a story that can be linked with the right brained activity of puzzling. For this exercise, the parent might use a picture story book for a young child or a regular story book for an older child, divide the book into segments or "parts", scramble them, and give the child the task of reassembling them in sensible order. This is training in using parts to create "whole thinking" and an illustration of how development in one sphere of the brain can be available and helpful to functioning on the other side of the brain.

It is usually not until the child reaches the upper grades and has to employ more part-whole type thinking before one notices that he may not be particularly good at this even though otherwise quite intelligent and with good basic academic skills. The upper grades in elementary school and, certainly, in middle school and high school and beyond require increasing perceptual-cognitive skills that involve a more whole-brain approach than simple basic reading skills acquisition, for instance. Thus, it behooves us to develop our children's right and left brain abilities insofar as possible.

PROCESSING SPEED

Speed of transfer of information from something seen (as, say, words or numbers in a book) to something written is one important form of processing. Another involves processing what is heard into instant action, as in taking lecture notes, for example. It is clearly an important skill in many academic and other areas.

Effective training in this area would include copying tasks using pencil and paper, card games such as Slap Jack, and Nintendo or other computer games that require quick reaction and the ability to shift focus rapidly. Such training develops a vigilant and responsive nervous system in the child though, clearly, if a child becomes overly excited by a particular form of stimulation, especially with Nintendo or arcade games, then it is probably best to limit the child's time with that activity or, in some instances, avoid using the activity. We want our children to have fine-tuned and quick nervous systems, but not hyperreactive or hyperactive ones.

NOTES

1. Gazzaniga, Michael. "The Split Brain In Man," *Scientific American*. August, 1967. pp. 24–29.
2. Ornstein, Robert. "The Split and Whole Brain," *Human Nature*, 1, 1978. pp. 76–83.
3. Springer, Sally and Deutsch, Georg. *Left Brain, Right Brain*. New York: Freeman. 1985. p. 236.
4. McCrone, John. *The Ape That Spoke: language and the evolution of the human mind*. New York: Morrow. 1991. p. 60.

5. Groth-Marnat, Gary. *Handbook of Psychological Assessment*. New York: Van Nostrad. 1984. p. 76.
6. Vitale, Barbara Meister. *Unicorns Are Real: a right brained approach to learning*. Rolling Hills Estates, CA: Jalmar Press. 1982. p. 51.

14

The Enhancement of Left Brain Thinking

The left brain is considered to be the center of the verbal, rational, linear and logical aspects of human cognition. The primary verbal cognitive skills involve:

- the ability to work with abstract symbols

- vocabulary

- verbal and visual memory, verbal fluency and general language skills

- knowledge of one's environment

- an informational base

- visual and auditory processing ability

Most of us want our children to function proficiently in these areas. For the most part, these are the areas of intelligence that tend to have great "payoff" value academically and, later, will extend into highly verbal careers such as attorneys, writers and psychotherapists, for example. Now it is time to focus on the various "domains" of verbal intelligence, what they are and how parents can assist in their enhancement.

GENERAL FUND OF INFORMATION

We all have general information stored in our memory. This information is not necessarily obtained in formal school lessons, or even
consciously. Rather, this general fund of data tends to be built upon
"incidental" or casual learning. Such learning takes place whether or
not the child, or the adult, is actually trying to master a skill or a body
of knowledge. Incidental learning just happens. We just come to
"know" (by being aware and listening to others) how to make hot
chocolate, or in which direction San Francisco is from Los Angeles, or
the name of a season, for example.

Some individuals obtain this kind of information much faster, and
have more of it, than others. This happens partly because of home
enrichment factors and school background. But the store of general
information also increases because of cognitive factors which appear
to be built into the child's developing brain. These include the power
of recall memory and the ability to be alert to many facets of one's
environment. Recall memory probably once played a vitally important part in helping our ancestors find their way to food and find their
way home again. Today such memory creates good *Trivial Pursuit*
players, of course, but also helps us remember where the nearest mail
box is, or recall a fragment of important information we have read in
an investment journal or scientific paper.

Children who do not have a rich store of general information about
the world in which they live, tend to be not particularly curious intellectually and not very interested in reading for pleasure. They are also apt to watch much television. In addition, they generally come from
families who do not spend much time engaged in activities such as
board games, reading, visiting museums, or discussing new ideas or
worldly issues.

Thus, to heighten your child's ability to gather and remember incidental information you must, as we've stated before, curtail TV,
spend time reading books (trips to the library or book store are vital)
and talking with the child as well as playing board games such as *Life,
Monopoly, Trivial Pursuit for Children, and Jeopardy*, for example.

If you personally do not enjoy these activities, yet feel that they are
important for your child, consider hiring an "enrichment tutor" (an
adult, possibly a teacher, who does like these activities and has some
grasp of what you are trying to do). Or you could look for other family members who might be pressed into service (grandparents; older
siblings) and who would welcome the opportunity to spend this kind
of focused time with the child.

Activities such as Scouting should be considered. The Boy Scouts and Girl Scouts deal with crafts, camping trips and outings which include much incidental learning of terrain, compass readings and so on. A Scout troop, however, is only as good as its leader so you need to do some research before you have your child join a troop.

Interest in sports can lead to much informational expansion as the parent extends the child's interest in a particular player or team and then extends this to broader aspects of geography (where the teams are) and interest in the stadiums and their history.

Also, children tend to identify with stars or well-known people. The child is in the process of defining himself so he may take on aspects of not only his parents or other relatives such as an admired older sibling but, also, bits of what he thinks a rock star's personality is, or aspects of a movie or television star. The alert and well-informed parent can build upon any of these interests and expand informational knowledge in countless ways.

For example, a girl might like ballet and want to become a ballerina. We expand on this interest, even though we are aware that the actual likelihood of any given person becoming a full-fledged ballerina is small. We can discuss The Nutcracker Suite, and go to see it as well as other ballets. We can enroll the child in ballet lessons and visit the library or book store for material on ballets and ballerinas. We can research the entire arena of ballet, which includes famous male and female dancers and many rich traditions.

Probably the single worst habit many adults have is talking too much in a "teaching-preaching" manner to young children. Exclamations of enjoyment are appropriate, of course, as are comments or even questions (not too many of these, however). As with many areas of child development, if you talk too much the child may turn off to you and this may ruin your potential for being the child's best tutor or coach in so many aspects of life.

ABSTRACT REASONING

Abstract reasoning at a basic level is finding the common elements between two things or ideas. To do such reasoning, the child must figure out how two things belong together or what conceptual classification they fit. For example, How are a dog and a rabbit alike? That they are both animals would be a good, high level response; the fact that they each have four legs, while correct, is not at as high a level of abstraction. The child must use inductive reasoning and move from particulars (dog and rabbit) to more general principles or rules of classification. The child must, of course, have had exposure to animals such as dogs and rabbits (and many other things as well), and be able to access his memory for the basic information while sorting out how this information can be developed into something more general that the two animals have in common.

An individual who cannot think well on an abstract level, may tend to think too literally. Academically, this could be a problem in the upper elementary grades, middle school and beyond since the subjects are often represented with high levels of symbolism and abstraction. The good abstract thinker tends to be able to more or less quickly perceive relationships or common threads among sometimes seemingly disparate elements.

To help your child develop the ability to perceive common relationships, you can ask questions which are almost pleasurable comments about aspects of the stores ("Look. Another knight. They all look alike in their armor, don't they? I just thought of something. I am thinking of an animal that has armor like a knight. Can you think of one like that?"). There are many examples to choose from. The idea is to get the child to start thinking about similarities between the elements in his world.

It may be that many children are far better abstract thinkers than they are given credit for. If we eavesdrop on or, better, engage in a discussion about sports, MTV, or social status with elementary school age children we often find some very high levels of abstract thinking. The basketball buffs can easily tell you the difference between the rough and ready play of the Knicks, for example, versus the less physical fast-break style of the Lakers. This same type of natural and informal abstraction is seen in other areas as the child compares rap with hard rock or some other form of music; regular board games versus Dungeons and Dragons, TV viewing with the interactive possibilities of CD-Roms or virtual reality arcade games.

In other words, many children have good abstract reasoning skills but don't realize this. Nor do their parents or teachers. This is often because of the way adults phrase something or ask a question such as, "How are these two things alike? How are they different?" Or in school the student may be asked to formally compare and contrast things. The problem at times is that the child's mind is often still functioning in an informal mode. So the child often feels he does not know the answer when, in fact, it is the structure of the question that confuses him.

As mentioned, gently pointing out how things are alike or different is useful. This will, hopefully, later lead to effective performance by the student on the "compare and contrast" questions often asked in upper school and college.

The parent needs to show the child that he often already has much information, that he can easily figure things out, and that you can prove this because he does it again and again when talking about sports, or MTV, or movie stars, or whomever and whatever. He needs to be told that he is a terrific abstract thinker because, within obvious limits, of course, most children really are.

RANGE OF VOCABULARY

Vocabulary level is considered to be one of the best general estimates of overall intelligence. The child's vocabulary reflects background factors such as education and her parents socioeconomic level. If the child's preschool years lacked educational stimulation, it is fortunate that her vocabulary level can be raised in the middle childhood years and beyond by reading and focused tutoring.

Reading and talking to your child are the initial best ways to enhance her vocabulary. We mentioned the benefits of reading before. You can read just about anything that you feel is appropriate to your child that she finds interesting. The *Read Aloud Handbook* by Jim Trelease has been mentioned before as a helpful guide. Your librarian or book store manager can also point you toward excellent material.

It is, of course, very easy to talk to your child. Parents do this every-day. When you are talking to your school age child, however, there is no need to hold back on your vocabulary. If you mean to say "under duress" or "attenuated" or "exacerbated," for example, then say it. With this age child, we are no longer using "motherese" as discussed earlier. Use all the words that are in your vocabulary to transmit them to the child in the context of conversational daily life. This will build her vocabulary quickly.

As we've stated before, you need to start reading to your child early and "hook" the child on stories. Also, make sure that what you read to your child is interesting and your voice is animated. Initially read for short periods of time, enough to whet the child's appetite and keep her coming back for more. If possible, end at an exciting or suspenseful part so that, like the old Saturday adventure serials, you have a story to come back to for the next reading.

Check the stores for computer games that can help build vocabulary. Word games such as *Scrabble* and *Junior Scrabble* help children exercise their knowledge of words, also.

STREET SMARTS

Practical judgment or "street smarts" is a highly useful form of intelligence throughout life. In developing this area, the child is asked what should you do if...type questions (What should you do if you see the sprinklers overflowing in your neighbor's yard?). Or, he is confronted with "why" type questions (Why do we have stop lights on some street corners?). It is important for children to know the what and why of rules and conventions in our society.

Children with good practical judgment often are judged brighter than those who are less well-developed in this area. This appears to be because these children are "savvy"; they just know how and why things appear to function in the real world. Some feel that street smarts or good judgment are innate, but I believe parents can help their child develop skill in this area through *training*.

As with any other type of training, we first need to break the overall task—the development of social judgment and practical knowledge—down into smaller bits and pieces. One of the smaller "bits" certainly would involve awareness and knowledge of social rules and regulations, which includes the reasons for traffic rules and regulations on behavior such as not passing gas or belching in the presence of others. When we stop to think about the teaching of such rules and regulations, we realize that most of these are informally transmitted to the child on an as-needed basis. This informal system tends to be quite efficient, for the most part, and generally gets most of the job done.

In addition to as-needed teaching, you can instruct through the use of games. These can be easily made up and fun to play while the two of you are driving in the car, sitting in the doctor's waiting room, or just hanging out while waiting for Nordstroms to open. These can be fanciful or serious. "What would you do if you saw Jasmine on a magic carpet in the parking lot of a store? If you were invited, where would you like to go with Jasmine?" You can ask, "What would you do if a person you didn't know asked you to take a ride in a car? What would you do if it's getting late and mom expects you home before dark?" You can vary this game by letting the child ask you similar questions, too.

When a child and parent become engaged in a game like this, the parent can often learn a good deal about the child's fears and fantasies. For instance, a child may ask questions regarding what would you do if you got divorced, or got fired from a job, or were not invited to an important wedding. If you get these kinds of questions, don't break off the game by dismissing, downplaying, or even directly reassuring the child that these things are not going to happen. Rather, answer the question straightforwardly but embed your answer with reassurances. ("Well, if we got divorced, which is very, very unlikely, I would try to remain on friendly terms with your father and we would both do our best to take good care of you since we love you).

Social training takes place implicitly and explicitly all the time, throughout the child's growing up years and beyond. Even as adults, when we go into new situations such as a new job, or getting to know your neighbor in a new town, or in the first stages of a new relationship, we know, from our past learning, to tread lightly and size up the situation for awhile.

Some children are "naturals" at perceiving and understanding how their environment works, both its social and mechanical aspects. Others just don't pick up subtle cues well and their behavior may, at times, be slightly out of synch with the expectations of others or even the rules of the school or team. When a friend comes over to play with your child, your child may need to be told to not wander off after a few minutes to play Nintendo by himself. If the child doesn't get it, you should help your child modify his behavior to become more socially appropriate.

A final note, it's best not to feel too uncomfortable if your child may not be perceiving the social nuances or other aspects of his environment. Many children don't perceive some of the problem areas of life very readily. That's why they need a great deal of training. That's what parents are for.

AUDITORY AND VISUAL ATTENTION SPAN

Auditory and visual attention span are obviously important as facilitators for the various domains of intelligence, and an argument could be made that these aspects of cognitive functioning are part of what we mean when we call a child "bright" or "alert." In any case, most parents and teachers would clearly prefer that their children's span of attention be longer rather than shorter. Television, with its rapid changing and shifting of visual and auditory images, undermines attention span. This is so even though parents say to me that their child must have a good attention span since he spends so much time in front of the TV, virtually without taking his eyes off the screen. As just noted, the TV images shift so rapidly that no attention span is required and the fact that the child remains glued to the screen is *not*, necessarily, a sign of a sustained span of attention.

Training for longer spans of concentration brings us back to activities such as reading or being read aloud to; construction of something through knitting or model making; quiet sustained conversation with a peer or adult; focused play with dolls, soldiers, blocks, Legos, crayons or other art materials. Concentration on music, the mastery of dance routines, and the practice of certain sports such as golf and games such as chess appear to enhance concentration abilities in specialized ways, though they may not generalize readily to other activities requiring sustained concentration such as academic work.

MATH AND COMPUTER SKILLS

The modern world requires individuals of high verbal, math or computer skills. The development of verbal skills has been discussed above. The development of math and computer skills is extremely important for the modern child.

Children who are literate in math, tend to be adept with computers. Almost all children, it appears, will soon have a personal computer available to them on which they will be able to write, compose music, create programs, perform spreadsheet and other basic data functions, and do math calculations faster than the greatest scientists of previous ages could ever do them. Young parents of today tend to be comfortable, in general, with computers. It is likely that they will introduce their children to the many facets of the computer when the child is quite young. And this is appropriate.

Computers can be excellent teachers. They are patient and even-tempered. Software teaching programs are constructed to repeat a problem when a mistake has been made, even dropping back to a previous lesson if necessary. The user is rewarded with a response such as a beep or encouraging word when the correct answer is selected. Parents should peruse software stores and subscribe to some of the new and excellent computer magazines for children (and for parents who have children).

Note: Parents need to be not only tutors, as has been urged throughout the book, but also *monitors* of what gets into their child's brain. GIGO is very operative in the world of material developed for sale to children—garbage in, garbage out. We are not going to get even close to the literacy of a Thomas Jefferson or the math adroitness of an Isaac Newton if we are allowing our children to interact with material more suitable for the mind-set of Attila the Hun.

Basic math at the elementary level builds toward math fluency and ease in the upper grades and in later life. Unfortunately, however, many of our children, for whatever reason, do not gain much proficiency in basic math. As can be easily observed at any fast food chain and many other places of business as well, clerks no longer have to make change in the way it once had to be done (counting out from the base price, redoing the calculation into your hand when giving back the change). Why don't clerks today have to do this? Most of them can't and, besides, the computerized cash register does it for them. Which came first, the register which could count change or the clerks who could not is difficult to say. But we can take note that many of today's children do not appear to be well-grounded in basic, everyday math. This is the math of common sense and daily life and, as some would agree, the most important math of all for most of us.

The elementary school age child needs to be exposed to numbers. She needs to learn how to count, add, subtract, divide, and multiply. She will need to master long division or, in the future, possibly not since many schools allow calculators to be used now. The concept of fractions should be mastered, as should the use of decimals. Children today seem to have difficulty with conversions such as feet to inches or minutes to hours (as in how many minutes in two and one half hours?). Many cannot find an average. Although this is taught in school, the fact that so many children just can't do it is a bit of a mystery. Possibly because, unlike words, they don't use the material of numbers and numerical concepts very much in their daily lives.

The child is used to answering questions from parents about what he did in school or what the movie was about. However, he is rarely asked what percentage of the class was absent that day, or what was the average score for the class on math test. A child probably isn't reminded, either that there are 12 items in a dozen, or 5,280 feet in a mile, or that Mt. Whitney is over 14,000 feet high with Mt. Everest being twice as high as that.

Briefly, to develop basic math skills we must find ways of working them into our daily lives. We all learn better from real life or concrete examples. When we read the morning sports pages with our child and note that a basketball player took the inbound pass, dribbled the length of the court, and made the winning basket in less than 4.8 seconds, how might the child interpret this? Is that fast or slow? How can we estimate how long 4.8 seconds is? How many seconds in a game? How fast is a nanosecond, do you suppose? What about light years?

In short, there are numbers all around us to be plucked out of our imaginations and used for the edification of ourselves and our children. All we have to do is think about it for awhile, use our imaginations, then set aside some time to teach our child. Providing the time seems to be the hardest part for most busy parents. We are going to address ourselves to that issue in the final chapter.

IV

PARENTS, GRANDPARENTS AND OTHER IMPORTANT PEOPLE

─── 15 ───

Grandparents and Other Important People Who can Help

It may not take a whole village to raise a child but a lot of involvement from many people sure does help. In our current hurried and fragmented times, busy parents, no matter how loving and caring, often just run out of time and energy before they can ever get into any kind of significant "cognitive enrichment" program as has been described in the preceding pages. There is just no getting around the fact, however, that any attempt to maximize your child's intelligence is going to be very labor-intensive (and, remember, this does not mean high pressure).

Low pressure, but labor-intensive. This means that the parent or some other trusted person must put in a lot of time with the child. This is a critical aspect of any cognitive development program. No television program, video or CD-ROM can do the job.

Busy parents, while usually desirous of spending time with their child, guiding her thinking, delighting in her joys and discoveries as she learns, simply do not have the time to do all that they might like to do. The truly loving and caring parents will quickly perceive that their child is in good hands, also, with grandparents or other relatives who live nearby. Grandparents, when available, are especially good resources. They usually have time, dote on the grandchild and tend to reinforce every "smart" thing they see the child do. Grandparents can provide mini-field trips about the city, including trips to the library, fire station, museums and so on.

Dr Arthur Kornhaber, a psychiatrist who created the Foundation for Grandparenting and who has authored two books on the subject, *Contemporary Grandparenting*[1] and *Grandparent Power!*,[2] states:

> Kids (who have frequent contact) with their grandparents are broader and deeper people. They have a sense of the past. They know other languages. They do better in school. They have a good sense of family and family values. Interestingly, they also have a sense of shame, which I think is disappearing from American children.[3]

However, young parents or new parents are sometimes reluctant to allow their child much time with anyone but themselves. Clearly, if the parents realized the value of a broad base of loving people who care for and teach a child, they would seek out "shared parenting" relationships for their children.

Grandparents must, of course, know their place and realize that they do not make decisions with respect to issues which should rightly be reserved for the parents. The child may be emotionally confused, even harmed, by the undermining of parental authority. Grandparents can and should, however, enrich the child's life intellectually and emotionally.

Two scenarios.

SCENARIO 1

A young mother gives birth to the child for whom she seems to have been waiting all her life. The child validates the mother's reason for existence and she is the center of the mother's life. The mother openly states that she lives through her child. Mother and daughter attend Mommy and Me classes, Gymboree classes, and any and all other gatherings of that type. This mother, however, finds it difficult to share her child with others, including caring grandparents.

She has a neurotic need to bind the child to her. Behind this is the fear of her child becoming attached to someone other than herself. This mother does not realize that love is an endless feast. No matter how you divide the pie, there is still plenty more. This is because love is expansive. The child becomes more capable of love the more she gets and gives love. This mother is actually shutting down her child's chances for increased cognitive stimulation from grandparents and others and, also, undermining the child's chances for the development of long-standing affectional relationships which are founded on an individual's basic sense of security.

SCENARIO 2

A young mother gives birth to her child whom she loves dearly. Because she is secure in her own sense of self, this mother is able to enjoy the fact that others love her child also. Indeed, she actively reaches out to grandparents and older friends, especially, to include them in the child's life. This child exists within a network of caring grandparents, relatives and older friends of the parents. In effect, because of the mother's care and skill in keeping in touch with many people, the child has two sets of loving grandparents as well as another set of surrogate grandparents and close involvement with uncles, aunts and other relatives. One is tempted to feel that real caring for a child involves much sharing of the child.

In the above scenarios, we spoke only of mother and daughter in order to simplify the story. In real life, of course, fathers are also involved (hopefully) and must assist the mother not only in rearing the child but, also, in support of her efforts to reach out and involve others in their and the child's life. Enrichment for the child does not come from attending classes, watching TV, or just sitting at home. Rather, enrichment, both intellectually and personally, derives from a myriad of positive interactions with others who love her and love her parents and who will spend kind and quiet time with her while introducing her to the many wonders of this world.

Most grandparents need little help from a book such as this one. They have raised their own children and they often seem to almost innately know how to spend positive, quality time with a child. This is probably because they are older and more experienced. Generally, they are not rushed. They can sit and talk, or take a walk. Or bake a cake. Spending quality time, it has been said, comes very close to looking like wasting time. Just hanging out and hanging around. Grandparents are a terrific resource and are great for slowing down the pace of life.

So, whether you, personally, get along with your parents or your mother-in-law or father-in-law, consider the fact that this may not be really important. What is really important is that they love your child, will be kind to her, will spend time with her, and will enhance her life.

And you do have something very important in common with them—love for your child.

NOTES

1. Kornhaber, Arthur. *Contemporary Grandparenting*. New York: Sage, 1996.
2. Kornhaber, Arthur. *Grandparent Power!* New York: Crown, 1994.
3. "Arthur Kornhaber: a few grandparenting lessons from America's most outspoken grandpa," *Modern Maturity*, January–February 1997: 53–71.3.

16

The Parent as Coach, Guide, Tutor and Role Model

Conceiving and giving birth to a child is easy compared to parenting. Also, it takes very little in the way of knowledge or even experience on the part of a mother or father to have a baby. On the other hand, it takes a great deal of time and thought to be a good parent. What exactly is a "good parent?"

Clearly, the good parent offers physical security to the child. The child cannot fend for himself (and, unlike the young of many other species will not be able to do so for many years) and the necessities of life—food and shelter, must be provided. In many ways, this is the easiest part of parenting.

All parents teach their children a great deal. This teaching can be judged to be negative when the child is taught that he is not a lovable individual, or he observes meanness and violence from parents, or he is taught that the world is a dangerous and fearful place and so on. The teaching can be positive when the child learns that he is regarded with respect, he is courteous and kind because his parents are courteous and kind to him, he feels wanted and loved and thus is able to like and love others. All these things and more, indeed, practically everything that we do and are, we learn from others in our culture. Parents are the backbone of the culture's dictates of what should or should not be done.

Many parents have commented about the difficulty of raising a child with values in a highly secularized society. They note that they are not particularly religious and, indeed, some are ambiguous about exposing their child to religious teaching of any kind since they feel that religions are hypocritical, based on myth, and often simply cause conflict. Of course, they admit, not being religious or, more to the point, not having any real value system can cause even more trouble. What is the answer?

I believe that one can and must teach values to children. To live "value free" is to be in a moral vacuum. However, the alternative is not, necessarily, to embrace one of the religions; it is dealing with the concepts of right and wrong, of good and evil. We need to teach our children that there really are "right ways" and "wrong ways" in life, that there really is good and evil. We don't necessarily need to be-lieve in the rewards of a Heaven or the punishment of a Hell in order to feel that there are right and wrong ways to treat one another and to live.

In a pinch, one could simply turn to what is termed in the *Boy Scout Handbook* the "Scout Law."[1] The Law is straightforward with respect to how an individual, in this case, a Scout, should conduct himself and straightforwardly advocates attributes such as trustworthiness, loyalty, friendliness, helpfulness, courtesy and kindness. Cleanliness, thriftiness and bravery are noted, as is reverence and respect for the beliefs of others.

If a parent taught those values, she couldn't go wrong. The reverence toward God, as I see it, is funneled into a spiritual reverence toward life that includes environmental and humanistic duties.

There are other values to be taught, of course, but the Scout Law offers a good start if one needs a framework. The parent must, of course, live by these values and these words, too. Actions do speak louder than words and it is hypocritical and essentially useless to talk morals and values to a child unless one lives them herself.

Note: As stated before, three words which should be heavily emphasized by all parents of all children as they assist their child in growing up are a simple "Please" and "Thank You."

A coach helps in skill development and in game strategy, the tutor offers one-on one-assistance, the guide helps us find our way and then not lose our path—all of these coalesce into parental love and help us as we seek to guide our children. The good parent uses these factors in a thoughtful and balanced manner to enhance the develop-ment of her child.

NOTE

1. Birkby, Robert C. *The Boy Scout Handbook, Tenth Edition.* Irving, Texas: Boy Scouts of America. 1990.

INDEX